I0702220

HODGKIN LYMPHOMA DIET COOKBOOK

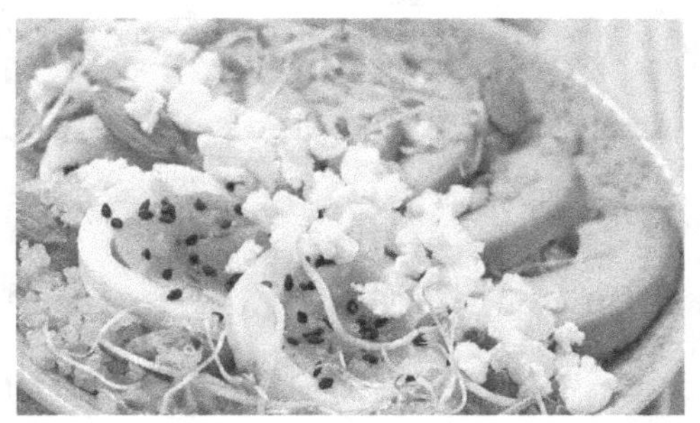

A Comprehensive Guide with Anti-Inflammatory Foods and Immune-Boosting Ingredients to Embrace a Healthy Approach to Eating for Recovery

KELLY C. BROWN

All rights reserved. No part of this publication may be reproduced, distributed, or transmitted in any form or by any means, including photocopying, recording, or other electronic or mechanical methods, without the prior written permission of the publisher, except in the case of brief quotations embodied in critical reviews and certain other noncommercial uses permitted by copyright law.

Copyright ©[Kelly C. Brown] 2024.

CONTENTS

INTRODUCTION

Clara's adventure began when she was diagnosed with Hodgkin lymphoma, a difficult and life-changing disease. Clara, determined to pursue all paths of healing, turned to a Hodgkin cancer diet cookbook advised by her nutritionist.

The cookbook stressed a holistic approach, emphasizing nutrient-dense foods with anti-inflammatory and immune-boosting characteristics. Clara adopted a diet rich in vibrant fruits and vegetables, lean proteins, and whole grains, all of which were thoroughly detailed in the cookbook's recipes.

Clara made her way through the suggested meal plans with steadfast dedication, integrating anti-cancer substances such as turmeric, ginger, and garlic. She learnt to prepare nutritious meals that aided her general health while addressing specific components of Hodgkin lymphoma.

Regular check-ups with her medical team revealed encouraging signs of recovery. Clara's commitment to the Hodgkin lymphoma diet not only aided her physical recovery, but it also gave her a sense of empowerment and control over her health.

Clara's health gradually improved, and she shared her success story with others suffering similar issues. The Hodgkin lymphoma diet cookbook became a significant resource for individuals looking for an alternative to conventional therapies.

Clara's journey underscored the potential of personalized, nutrient-focused diets in supporting health and recovery. Her story inspired many to explore the intersection of nutrition and healing, demonstrating that a well-crafted diet could be a crucial component of a comprehensive approach to managing and overcoming serious health conditions.

Welcome to the "Nourish & Thrive: Hodgkin Lymphoma Diet Cookbook," a culinary guide to help individuals on their path to wellness. This cookbook, created with care and informed by nutritional experience, is an invaluable resource for anyone living with Hodgkin Lymphoma.

CHAPTER 1: UNDERSTANDING HODGKIN LYMPHOMA

Hodgkin lymphoma, also known as Hodgkin disease, is a kind of cancer that affects the lymphatic system, which is an important component of your immune system. By filtering and transmitting white blood cells termed lymphocytes, this network of arteries and nodes aids in the fight against infection and disease. These cells begin to proliferate abnormally in Hodgkin lymphoma, creating tumors within the lymph nodes and potentially spreading throughout the body.

Important Information About Hodgkin Lymphoma:

- Relatively uncommon: Hodgkin lymphoma is uncommon in comparison to other malignancies, accounting for roughly 1% of all new cancer diagnoses each year.

- Affects people of all ages: While Hodgkin lymphoma can occur at any age, it is more frequent in young adults between the ages of 15 and 40, as well as those over the age of 55.

- There are two primary types: The two primary kinds are classic Hodgkin lymphoma and nodular lymphocyte-predominant Hodgkin lymphoma (NLPHL), which are distinguished by their microscopic appearance and therapeutic approaches.
- Treatment and cure: Hodgkin lymphoma, fortunately, is one of the most treatable and curable types of cancer, with high success rates depending on parameters such as stage and type.

Symptoms:

Because early detection is critical for effective treatment, being aware of potential signs is critical. These could include:

- Swollen lymph nodes that are painless and usually located in the neck, armpit, or groin, but can occur anywhere.
- Fever: An unexplained and persistent fever, sometimes accompanied by nocturnal sweats.
- Weight loss that is unexplained: Loss of 10% or more of body weight in 6 months.
- Fatigue is defined as persistent and inexplicable fatigue.

- Itchy skin: This is most common after bathing or drinking alcohol.
- Other symptoms include chest pain, shortness of breath, difficulty sleeping, and a cough.

Causes and risk factors include:

Although the actual cause of Hodgkin lymphoma is unknown, the following factors may raise the risk:

- Epstein-Barr virus (EBV): EBV infection is associated with an elevated risk, although most infected people do not acquire the disease.
- Family history: Having a family member with Hodgkin lymphoma raises your risk marginally.
- Immune system weakness: HIV/AIDS or immunosuppressive drugs can increase the risk.

Diagnosis and Treatment:

Physical examination, blood tests, imaging scans, biopsy, and bone marrow aspiration are all used to make a diagnosis. Individual characteristics such as stage, type, and overall health influence treatment plans. Treatment options that are commonly used include:

- Chemotherapy is the use of powerful medications to kill cancer cells.

- Radiation therapy: The use of focused radiation beams to kill cancer cells.

- Stem cell transplantation is the process of replacing bone marrow that has been damaged by treatment with healthy donor cells.

- Balanced diet: A well-balanced diet promotes general well-being and will help to boost your immune system.

IMPORTANCE OF NUTRITION IN MANAGING HODGKIN LYMPHOMA

Nutrition is critical in the treatment of Hodgkin Lymphoma, and a specific dietary strategy, such as that indicated in this Hodgkin Lymphoma Diet Cookbook, can have a substantial impact on the well-being and rehabilitation of those dealing with this difficult condition.

1. Immune Support: Adequate nutrition is necessary for maintaining a strong immune system, which is critical in the battle against malignant cells. This cookbook features meals high in vitamins, minerals, and antioxidants, which boost immune function and the body's natural defense systems.

2. Dealing with Treatment Side Effects: Cancer therapies, such as chemotherapy and radiation therapy, frequently have side effects that affect appetite, taste, and nutrient absorption. This Hodgkin Lymphoma Diet Cookbook includes dishes intended to ease these side effects, such as providing easily digestible and appetizing meals to minimize malnutrition while undergoing treatment.

3. Keeping Your Weight and Energy Levels Up: Cancer and its therapies can cause weight loss, muscle atrophy, and weariness. This cookbook includes recipes that emphasize nutrient density and calorie content, so assisting individuals in maintaining or regaining a healthy weight and energy levels.

4. Inflammation Reduction: Chronic inflammation has been linked to cancer progression. A well-planned diet, as stated in this cookbook, includes anti-inflammatory foods like omega-3 fatty acids, turmeric, and ginger, which may benefit in inflammation management and overall well-being.

5. Psychological Well-Being: A well-rounded nutritional approach covers both physical and psychological components of the journey. Delicious, wholesome meals from the cookbook can improve mood and provide a sense of control and comfort during a difficult period.

FOODS TO EAT AND FOODS TO AVOID

FOODS TO EAT

1. Colorful fruits and vegetables: High in vitamins, minerals, and antioxidants, these foods help the immune system and supply critical nutrients for overall health. Include a wide range of colors to ensure a broad range of benefits.

2. Whole Grains: Choose whole grains such as brown rice, quinoa, and whole wheat for fiber, vitamins, and minerals. Fiber promotes digestion and helps to maintain consistent energy levels.

3. Lean Protein: Choose fowl, fish, beans, and lentils as lean protein sources. Protein is essential for muscle health and regeneration, and this is especially important during cancer therapy.

4. Healthy Fats: Include avocados, almonds, seeds, and olive oil as sources of healthy fats. These fats provide long-lasting energy and promote general wellness.

5. Tumeric and Ginger: Turmeric and ginger have anti-inflammatory effects and may aid in the management of inflammation associated with Hodgkin Lymphoma. Include them in your recipes for flavor as well as potential health advantages.

6. High-Calorie, Nutrient-Dense Foods: Use calorie-dense foods like smoothies, nut butters, and energy-dense snacks to combat weight loss and exhaustion. These can assist in meeting nutritional requirements despite probable appetite fluctuations.

7. Beverages for Hydration: Stay hydrated by drinking water, herbal teas, and clear broths. Proper hydration is essential for general health and can help with the management of certain therapeutic side effects.

FOODS TO AVOID

1. Processed and Refined Foods: Limit your intake of processed and refined foods, which generally lack nutritional value and may contribute to inflammation.

2. Added Sugars: Limit your intake of foods and beverages containing added sugars. High sugar consumption can have an impact on energy levels and general health.

3. Foods that are fried or high in fat: While healthy fats are helpful, eating too many fried and high-fat foods can lead to weight gain. Consume healthy fats in moderation.

4. Foods High in Sodium: Limit your sodium consumption by avoiding highly processed and salty foods. This aids in the management of fluid retention, which is a potential side effect of some medications.

5. Alcohol: Limit or avoid alcohol drinking because it can interfere with certain drugs and jeopardize overall health.

6. Raw Seafood and Undercooked Meats: Avoiding raw or undercooked fish and meats is a good way to practice food safety. This lowers the chance of infections, which can be difficult to manage during cancer therapy.

7. Caffeine: While moderate caffeine consumption is normally safe, excessive caffeine consumption can lead to dehydration. Keep an eye on your overall hydration consumption.

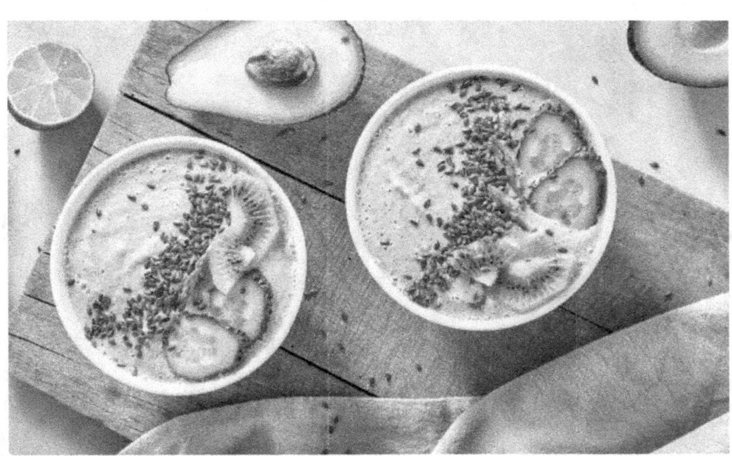

"I nourish my body with
wholesome, healing foods
to support my journey to
wellness."

"Every meal I prepare is a
step towards
strengthening my body
and boosting my immune
system."

CHAPTER 2: HODGKIN LYMPHOMA SHOPPING LIST

A diet for individuals with Hodgkin lymphoma should focus on promoting overall health, supporting the immune system, and managing potential side effects of treatment.

Here's a shopping list that includes a variety of nutrient-rich foods:

1. **Fruits and Vegetables:**
   - Berries (blueberries, strawberries, raspberries)
   - Citrus fruits (oranges, grapefruits, lemons)
   - Dark leafy greens (spinach, kale, Swiss chard)
   - Cruciferous vegetables (broccoli, cauliflower, Brussels sprouts)
   - Avocado
   - Sweet potatoes
   - Bell peppers
2. **Whole Grains:**
   - Quinoa

- Brown rice
- Whole wheat pasta
- Oats
- Barley
- Farro

3. **Lean Proteins:**
   - Skinless poultry (chicken, turkey)
   - Fish (salmon, tuna, trout)
   - Legumes (beans, lentils, chickpeas)
   - Tofu and tempeh
   - Eggs

4. **Healthy Fats:**
   - Olive oil
   - Avocado oil
   - Nuts (almonds, walnuts, pistachios)
   - Seeds (flaxseeds, chia seeds, sunflower seeds)

5. **Dairy or Dairy Alternatives:**
   - Low-fat or Greek yogurt
   - Milk fortified with vitamin D
   - Cheese (in moderation)
   - Dairy alternatives (almond milk, soy milk)

6. **Hydration:**
   - Water
   - Herbal teas
   - Coconut water
   - Broth-based soups
7. **Antioxidant-Rich Foods:**
   - Green tea
   - Colorful vegetables and fruits
   - Dark chocolate (in moderation)
8. **Ginger and Turmeric:**
   - Fresh ginger and turmeric for their anti-inflammatory properties
9. **Soft Foods:**
   - Mashed potatoes
   - Smoothies
   - Soups and stews

EATING OUT ON THE HODGKIN LYMPHOMA

Dining out can be difficult while following a Hodgkin Lymphoma diet, but with careful selections, it is feasible to maintain a healthful and supportive approach to managing the condition.

When dining out, keep the following things in mind:

1. Lean Proteins: Choose lean protein sources such grilled chicken, fish, or tofu. These options give needed protein without a lot of saturated fat, which is good for your general health.

2. Colorful veggies: Include a variety of colorful veggies to ensure a wide range of nutrients. Salads, veggie sides, and grilled vegetables are also options. These alternatives provide vitamins, minerals, and antioxidants that are essential for immune system support.

3. Choose Whole Grains: When it comes to carbohydrates, choose whole grains such as brown rice, quinoa, or whole wheat. When compared to processed grains, these grains deliver more fiber and minerals, encouraging digestive health.

4. Limit Processed Foods: Limit processed foods and high-sodium dishes. Reducing salt intake can help with fluid retention, which is a concern for some people with Hodgkin Lymphoma.

5. Keep an eye on portion sizes: To avoid overeating, keep portion proportions in mind. Consider ordering appetizers as a main entrée or sharing dishes. This method allows you to limit your calorie consumption while still enjoying a variety of flavors.

6. Maintain Adequate Hydration: Adequate hydration is critical. Instead of sugary drinks or excessive caffeine, drink water or herbal teas. Proper hydration promotes general well-being and aids in the management of probable therapeutic side effects.

7. Be Aware of Dietary limits: If you have special dietary limits owing to treatment side effects or other health concerns, tell them to the restaurant staff clearly. Many restaurants are willing to accommodate particular dietary requirements.

8. Moderate Sugar Consumption: Reduce your intake of sugary treats and beverages. While it is acceptable to indulge on occasion, eating a balanced diet with limited sugar intake is essential for general health.

9. Select foods produced Using Healthy Cooking Methods: Preferably choose foods produced using healthy cooking methods such as grilling, steaming, or baking. These approaches aid in retaining the nutritional content of foods while avoiding the addition of excessive fats.

10. Request alterations: Do not be afraid to request alterations to match your dietary needs. Most restaurants are willing to tailor dishes to personal preferences or dietary constraints.

7-DAY MEAL PLAN

Day 1:

Breakfast: Quinoa porridge with berries and almonds

Ingredients:
- 1 cup quinoa
- 2 cups water
- 2 cups milk (dairy or plant-based)
- 1/4 cup sliced almonds

- 1 cup mixed berries (strawberries, blueberries, raspberries)
- 2 tablespoons honey or maple syrup
- 1 teaspoon vanilla extract
- Pinch of salt

Instructions:

1. Rinse the quinoa thoroughly under cold water to remove any bitterness.
2. In a medium-sized saucepan, combine the rinsed quinoa and water. Bring it to a boil, then reduce the heat to low, cover, and simmer for about 15 minutes, or until the quinoa is cooked and the water is absorbed.
3. In a separate small pan, toast the sliced almonds over medium heat until they turn golden brown. Keep a close eye on them to prevent burning.
4. Once the quinoa is cooked, add the milk to the saucepan. Stir in the vanilla extract and a pinch of salt. Simmer on low heat for an additional 10-15 minutes, or until the porridge reaches your desired consistency.
5. While the porridge is cooking, wash and prepare the berries.

6. Once the porridge is ready, spoon it into serving bowls. Top each bowl with a generous handful of mixed berries and the toasted almonds.

7. Drizzle honey or maple syrup over the quinoa porridge for sweetness. Adjust the sweetness according to your taste.

8. Serve the quinoa porridge warm and enjoy your delicious and nutritious breakfast!

Lunch: Grilled salmon with steamed broccoli and sweet potato

Ingredients:

- 4 salmon filets
- 2 tablespoons olive oil
- 2 tablespoons lemon juice
- 2 cloves garlic, minced
- 1 teaspoon dried oregano
- Salt and pepper to taste

For steamed broccoli:

- 4 cups broccoli florets
- 1 tablespoon olive oil
- Salt and pepper to taste

For sweet potatoes:

- 2 large sweet potatoes, peeled and diced

- 2 tablespoons olive oil
- 1 teaspoon paprika
- Salt and pepper to taste

Instructions:

1. Preheat the grill to medium-high heat.

2. In a small bowl, whisk together olive oil, lemon juice, minced garlic, dried oregano, salt, and pepper to create the marinade for the salmon.

3. Place the salmon filets in a shallow dish and pour the marinade over them. Let it marinate for at least 15-30 minutes, allowing the flavors to infuse.

4. While the salmon is marinating, prepare the sweet potatoes. In a bowl, toss the diced sweet potatoes with olive oil, paprika, salt, and pepper. Spread them on a baking sheet.

5. Preheat the oven to 400°F (200°C) and roast the sweet potatoes for 20-25 minutes or until they are tender and lightly browned.

6. For the steamed broccoli, heat olive oil in a steamer or a pot with a steamer basket. Steam the broccoli for about 5-7 minutes until it's tender but still vibrant green. Season with salt and pepper.

7. Grill the marinated salmon filets on the preheated grill for about 4-5 minutes per side or until the fish flakes easily with a fork.

8. Assemble the plates by placing a grilled salmon filet alongside a serving of steamed broccoli and roasted sweet potatoes.

9. Garnish with additional lemon wedges and fresh herbs if desired.

10. Serve immediately, and enjoy your delicious and nutritious grilled salmon with steamed broccoli and sweet potatoes!

Snack: Greek yogurt with honey and walnuts

Ingredients:

- 1 cup Greek yogurt
- 2 tablespoons honey (adjust to taste)
- 1/4 cup chopped walnuts

Instructions:

1. Start by spooning the Greek yogurt into a serving bowl. Greek yogurt works well for this recipe because of its thick and creamy texture.

2. Drizzle honey over the Greek yogurt. Begin with 1-2 tablespoons and adjust according to your desired level of sweetness.

3. Take the chopped walnuts and sprinkle them evenly over the yogurt and honey mixture. Walnuts add a delightful crunch and nutty flavor.

4. Gently stir the ingredients together, ensuring that the honey and walnuts are evenly distributed throughout the yogurt.

5. You can choose to serve the Greek yogurt immediately or let it sit in the refrigerator for a short while to allow the flavors to meld.

6. Before serving, you might want to garnish with additional walnuts for a decorative touch.

7. Enjoy this simple and delicious Greek yogurt with honey and walnuts as a nutritious breakfast, snack, or dessert!

Dinner: Lentil soup with a side of mixed green salad

Ingredients for Lentil Soup:

- 1 cup dry green or brown lentils, rinsed and drained
- 1 onion, finely chopped

- 2 carrots, diced
- 2 celery stalks, diced
- 3 cloves garlic, minced
- 1 can (14 oz) diced tomatoes
- 6 cups vegetable or chicken broth
- 1 teaspoon ground cumin
- 1 teaspoon ground coriander
- 1/2 teaspoon smoked paprika
- Salt and pepper to taste
- 2 tablespoons olive oil
- Fresh lemon wedges (for serving)

Ingredients for Mixed Green Salad:

- 4 cups mixed salad greens (e.g., spinach, arugula, lettuce)
- 1 cucumber, sliced
- 1 cup cherry tomatoes, halved
- 1/4 red onion, thinly sliced
- 1/4 cup feta cheese, crumbled (optional)

For Salad Dressing:

- 3 tablespoons extra virgin olive oil
- 1 tablespoon balsamic vinegar
- 1 teaspoon Dijon mustard
- Salt and pepper to taste

Instructions for Lentil Soup:

1. In a large pot, heat olive oil over medium heat. Add chopped onions, carrots, and celery. Sauté until the vegetables are softened, about 5-7 minutes.
2. Add minced garlic, ground cumin, ground coriander, and smoked paprika to the pot. Cook for an additional 1-2 minutes until fragrant.
3. Pour in the rinsed lentils, diced tomatoes (with their juice), and broth. Bring the mixture to a boil, then reduce the heat to low, cover, and simmer for about 25-30 minutes or until the lentils are tender.
4. Season the lentil soup with salt and pepper to taste. Adjust the seasoning as needed.
5. Serve the lentil soup hot, with a squeeze of fresh lemon juice.

Instructions for Mixed Green Salad:

1. In a large bowl, combine the mixed salad greens, sliced cucumber, cherry tomatoes, and thinly sliced red onion.

2. In a small bowl or jar, whisk together the extra virgin olive oil, balsamic vinegar, Dijon mustard, salt, and pepper to create the salad dressing.
3. Drizzle the dressing over the salad and toss gently to coat the ingredients evenly.
4. If desired, sprinkle crumbled feta cheese over the salad for added flavor.
5. Serve the mixed green salad alongside the lentil soup for a balanced and wholesome meal.

Day 2:

Breakfast: Chia seed pudding with mango and kiwi

Ingredients:
For Chia Seed Pudding:
- 1/4 cup chia seeds
- 1 cup almond milk (or any milk of your choice)
- 1-2 tablespoons maple syrup or honey (adjust to taste)
- 1/2 teaspoon vanilla extract

For Mango and Kiwi Topping:

- 1 ripe mango, peeled and diced
- 2 kiwis, peeled and sliced

Optional Garnish:

- Fresh mint leaves

Instructions:

1. In a bowl, combine chia seeds, almond milk, maple syrup (or honey), and vanilla extract. Stir well to make sure the chia seeds are evenly distributed. Let it sit for a few minutes.

2. After a few minutes, stir the chia seed mixture again to prevent clumping. Cover the bowl and refrigerate it for at least 2 hours, or preferably overnight. The chia seeds will absorb the liquid and create a pudding-like consistency.

3. While the chia pudding is setting, prepare the fruit toppings. Peel and dice the ripe mango and slice the kiwis.

4. Once the chia pudding has reached the desired consistency, give it a good stir. If it's too thick, you can add a little more almond milk to reach your preferred thickness.

5. Spoon the chia seed pudding into serving glasses or bowls.

6. Top the chia pudding with the diced mango and sliced kiwi.

7. Optionally, garnish with fresh mint leaves for a burst of freshness.

8. Serve the chia seed pudding with mango and kiwi immediately, or refrigerate until ready to serve.

Lunch: Turkey and vegetable stir-fry with brown rice

Ingredients:

For Turkey and Vegetable Stir-Fry:

- 1 lb (about 450g) turkey breast, thinly sliced
- 2 tablespoons soy sauce
- 1 tablespoon oyster sauce
- 1 tablespoon hoisin sauce
- 1 tablespoon cornstarch
- 2 tablespoons vegetable oil, divided
- 3 cloves garlic, minced
- 1 tablespoon ginger, grated
- 1 red bell pepper, thinly sliced
- 1 yellow bell pepper, thinly sliced
- 1 cup broccoli florets
- 1 medium carrot, julienned

- 1 cup snow peas, ends trimmed
- 4 green onions, sliced (for garnish)
- Sesame seeds (optional, for garnish)

For Brown Rice:

- 1 cup brown rice
- 2 cups water
- 1/2 teaspoon salt

Instructions:

For Brown Rice:

1. Rinse the brown rice under cold water. In a saucepan, combine the rinsed rice, water, and salt.
2. Bring the rice to a boil, then reduce the heat to low, cover, and simmer for about 40-45 minutes or until the rice is tender and water is absorbed.
3. Once cooked, fluff the brown rice with a fork and set aside.

For Turkey and Vegetable Stir-Fry:

1. In a bowl, mix the thinly sliced turkey with soy sauce, oyster sauce, hoisin sauce, and cornstarch. Allow the turkey to marinate for about 15-20 minutes.

2. Heat 1 tablespoon of vegetable oil in a large wok or skillet over medium-high heat. Add the marinated turkey and stir-fry until it's cooked through. Remove the turkey from the wok and set it aside.

3. In the same wok, add another tablespoon of vegetable oil. Stir in minced garlic and grated ginger, cooking for about 30 seconds until fragrant.

4. Add sliced red and yellow bell peppers, broccoli florets, julienned carrots, and snow peas to the wok. Stir-fry the vegetables for 3-5 minutes until they are crisp-tender.

5. Return the cooked turkey to the wok and toss everything together until well combined and heated through.

6. Serve the turkey and vegetable stir-fry over the cooked brown rice.

7. Garnish with sliced green onions and sesame seeds if desired.

8. Enjoy your tasty and nutritious turkey and vegetable stir-fry with brown rice!

Snack: Fresh fruit salad with a sprinkle of flaxseeds

Ingredients:

- 2 cups mixed fresh fruits (such as strawberries, blueberries, grapes, pineapple, melon, and kiwi), washed and chopped
- 1 tablespoon honey or maple syrup (optional, for added sweetness)
- 1 tablespoon fresh lime or lemon juice
- 1-2 tablespoons ground flaxseeds

Instructions:

1. Wash, peel, and chop the desired fruits into bite-sized pieces. Choose a variety of fruits for a colorful and flavorful salad.
2. In a large mixing bowl, combine the mixed fresh fruits.
3. Drizzle honey or maple syrup over the fruits if you desire a sweeter taste. Add fresh lime or lemon juice for a hint of citrusy brightness.
4. Gently toss the fruits to ensure they are evenly coated with the sweetener and citrus juice.
5. Sprinkle ground flaxseeds over the fruit mixture. Flaxseeds add a nutty flavor and provide a boost of omega-3 fatty acids and fiber.

6. Toss the fruit salad again to distribute the flaxseeds evenly.

7. Let the fruit salad sit for a few minutes to allow the flavors to meld.

8. Serve the fresh fruit salad in individual bowls or on a platter.

9. Optionally, garnish with mint leaves for a refreshing touch.

10. Enjoy this healthy and vibrant fresh fruit salad with a sprinkle of flaxseeds!

Dinner: Baked chicken breast with quinoa and roasted Brussels sprouts

Ingredients:

For Baked Chicken Breast:

- 4 boneless, skinless chicken breasts
- 2 tablespoons olive oil
- 2 teaspoons garlic powder
- 2 teaspoons onion powder
- 1 teaspoon paprika
- 1 teaspoon dried thyme
- Salt and pepper to taste

For Quinoa:

- 1 cup quinoa, rinsed

- 2 cups chicken broth or water
- Salt to taste

For Roasted Brussels Sprouts:

- 1 pound Brussels sprouts, trimmed and halved
- 2 tablespoons olive oil
- Salt and pepper to taste

Instructions:

Baked Chicken Breast:

1. Preheat the oven to 400°F (200°C).
2. In a small bowl, mix together olive oil, garlic powder, onion powder, paprika, dried thyme, salt, and pepper to create a seasoning blend.
3. Place the chicken breasts on a baking sheet lined with parchment paper or lightly greased.
4. Brush the chicken breasts with the prepared seasoning blend, ensuring they are well coated on both sides.
5. Bake in the preheated oven for 20-25 minutes or until the internal temperature reaches 165°F (74°C) and the chicken is golden brown.

Quinoa:

1. While the chicken is baking, rinse the quinoa under cold water.

2. In a medium saucepan, combine quinoa and chicken broth (or water). Bring to a boil, then reduce heat to low, cover, and simmer for about 15 minutes, or until quinoa is cooked and liquid is absorbed.

Roasted Brussels Sprouts:

1. Preheat the oven to 400°F (200°C).
2. In a bowl, toss Brussels sprouts with olive oil, salt, and pepper until evenly coated.
3. Spread the Brussels sprouts on a baking sheet in a single layer.
4. Roast in the preheated oven for 20-25 minutes or until the Brussels sprouts are golden brown and crispy on the edges.

Assembling the Dish:

1. Arrange a bed of cooked quinoa on serving plates.
2. Place a baked chicken breast on top of the quinoa.
3. Serve with a generous portion of roasted Brussels sprouts on the side.
4. Optionally, garnish with fresh herbs like parsley or a drizzle of olive oil.

Day 3:

Breakfast: Smoothie with spinach, banana, berries, and a scoop of protein powder

Ingredients:

- 1 ripe banana
- 1 cup fresh or frozen mixed berries (strawberries, blueberries, raspberries)
- 2 cups fresh spinach leaves
- 1 scoop vanilla or unflavored protein powder
- 1 cup unsweetened almond milk (or any preferred milk)
- 1 tablespoon chia seeds (optional)
- Ice cubes (optional)

Instructions:

1. Peel the ripe banana and place it in the blender.
2. Add the mixed berries to the blender. If using fresh berries, you can also include a handful of ice cubes to make the smoothie colder.

3. Add the fresh spinach leaves to the blender. Spinach is a nutrient-packed addition that adds vitamins and minerals without overpowering the flavor.

4. Scoop in the protein powder of your choice. Vanilla-flavored powder complements the fruit flavors well.

5. Pour in the almond milk to the blender. Adjust the amount based on your desired thickness.

6. Optionally, add chia seeds for an extra boost of fiber and omega-3 fatty acids. Chia seeds also add a delightful texture to the smoothie.

7. Blend all the ingredients until smooth and creamy. If the smoothie is too thick, you can add more almond milk, a little at a time, until you reach your desired consistency.

8. Taste the smoothie and adjust sweetness if needed. If you prefer a sweeter smoothie, you can add a drizzle of honey or a few drops of vanilla extract.

9. Once well blended, pour the smoothie into glasses and enjoy immediately.

Lunch: Quinoa salad with chickpeas, cucumber, and cherry tomatoes

Ingredients:

- 1 cup quinoa, rinsed
- 2 cups water or vegetable broth
- 1 can (15 oz) chickpeas, drained and rinsed
- 1 cucumber, diced
- 1 cup cherry tomatoes, halved
- 1/2 red onion, finely chopped
- 1/4 cup fresh parsley, chopped
- 1/4 cup fresh mint, chopped (optional)
- 1/3 cup feta cheese, crumbled (optional)
- 3 tablespoons olive oil
- 2 tablespoons lemon juice
- 1 teaspoon ground cumin
- Salt and pepper to taste

Instructions:

1. In a medium saucepan, combine quinoa and water (or vegetable broth). Bring to a boil, then reduce heat to low, cover, and simmer for about 15 minutes, or until quinoa is cooked and water is absorbed. Fluff the quinoa with a fork and let it cool.

2. In a large mixing bowl, combine the cooked quinoa, drained chickpeas, diced cucumber, cherry tomatoes, chopped red onion, fresh parsley, and mint (if using).

3. In a small bowl, whisk together olive oil, lemon juice, ground cumin, salt, and pepper to create the dressing.

4. Pour the dressing over the quinoa mixture and toss everything together until well coated.

5. If using, sprinkle crumbled feta cheese over the salad and gently toss.

6. Taste the salad and adjust the seasoning or add more lemon juice if desired.

7. Chill the quinoa salad in the refrigerator for at least 30 minutes to allow the flavors to meld.

8. Before serving, give the salad a final toss and garnish with additional fresh herbs if desired.

Snack: Almond butter on whole-grain crackers

Ingredients:

- Whole-grain crackers
- Almond butter

Instructions:

1. Take whole-grain crackers of your choice and arrange them on a serving plate or tray.

2. Using a butter knife or a spoon, spread a generous layer of almond butter onto each cracker. Ensure an even coating for a balanced flavor.

3. Optional: You can drizzle a touch of honey or sprinkle a pinch of cinnamon on top of the almond butter for added sweetness and flavor.

4. Arrange the almond butter-covered crackers neatly on the serving plate.

5. Serve and enjoy these almond butter on whole-grain crackers as a tasty and nutritious snack!

Dinner: Grilled shrimp with asparagus and wild rice

Ingredients:

- 1 pound large shrimp, peeled and deveined
- 1 bunch fresh asparagus, trimmed
- 1 cup wild rice
- 2 tablespoons olive oil
- 3 cloves garlic, minced

- 1 lemon, juiced and zested
- Salt and pepper to taste
- 1 teaspoon paprika
- Fresh parsley, chopped (for garnish)

Instructions:

1. Cook the wild rice according to package instructions. Usually, it involves rinsing the rice, bringing it to a boil, and then simmering until tender. Set aside.
2. Preheat your grill to medium-high heat.
3. In a bowl, combine the shrimp with olive oil, minced garlic, lemon juice, lemon zest, salt, pepper, and paprika. Toss well to coat the shrimp evenly.
4. Thread the marinated shrimp onto skewers, alternating with asparagus spears.
5. Place the shrimp and asparagus skewers on the preheated grill. Grill for 2-3 minutes per side, or until the shrimp turn pink and opaque, and the asparagus is tender-crisp. Be cautious not to overcook.
6. While grilling, you can brush the skewers with any remaining marinade for added flavor.

7. Once the shrimp and asparagus are done, remove them from the grill.

8. Serve the grilled shrimp and asparagus over a bed of cooked wild rice.

9. Garnish with fresh chopped parsley and additional lemon wedges if desired.

10. Enjoy your delicious and healthy grilled shrimp with asparagus and wild rice!

Day 4:

Breakfast: Oatmeal with sliced apples, cinnamon, and a drizzle of honey

Ingredients:
- 1 cup old-fashioned rolled oats
- 2 cups water or milk (dairy or plant-based)
- 1 apple, cored and thinly sliced
- 1 teaspoon ground cinnamon
- 2 tablespoons honey
- Optional toppings: chopped nuts, raisins, or yogurt

Instructions:
1. In a saucepan, bring water or milk to a boil.

2. Stir in the rolled oats and reduce the heat to medium-low. Cook the oats, stirring occasionally, until they reach your desired consistency. This usually takes about 5-7 minutes.

3. While the oats are cooking, heat a small skillet over medium heat. Add the apple slices and sprinkle them with cinnamon. Sauté the apples until they are tender, about 3-5 minutes.

4. Once the oats are cooked, remove the saucepan from heat.

5. Transfer the cooked oats to a bowl. Top them with the sautéed apple slices.

6. Drizzle honey over the oatmeal and apples. Use more or less honey according to your sweetness preference.

7. Optional: Add additional toppings like chopped nuts, raisins, or a dollop of yogurt for extra texture and flavor.

8. Give everything a gentle stir to combine the ingredients.

9. Serve the oatmeal warm and enjoy a comforting and nutritious breakfast!

Lunch: Vegetable and lentil curry with whole-grain naan bread

Ingredients:

For the Curry:

- 1 cup dry lentils (red or green), rinsed and drained
- 2 tablespoons vegetable oil
- 1 onion, finely chopped
- 3 cloves garlic, minced
- 1 tablespoon ginger, grated
- 1 tablespoon curry powder
- 1 teaspoon ground cumin
- 1 teaspoon ground coriander
- 1 teaspoon turmeric
- 1 teaspoon paprika
- 1 can (14 oz) diced tomatoes
- 1 can (14 oz) coconut milk
- 3 cups mixed vegetables (e.g., carrots, bell peppers, peas, and spinach)
- Salt and pepper to taste
- Fresh cilantro, chopped (for garnish)

For the Whole-Grain Naan Bread:

- 2 cups whole wheat flour
- 1 teaspoon baking powder

- 1/2 teaspoon baking soda
- 1/4 teaspoon salt
- 1 cup plain yogurt
- 2 tablespoons olive oil
- 1 garlic clove, minced (optional, for garlic naan)

Instructions:

For the Curry:

1. Cook the lentils according to package instructions. Set aside.
2. In a large pot or deep skillet, heat the vegetable oil over medium heat. Add chopped onions and cook until softened.
3. Add minced garlic and grated ginger to the onions, sautéing for an additional minute until fragrant.
4. Stir in the curry powder, ground cumin, ground coriander, turmeric, and paprika. Cook the spices for 1-2 minutes to release their flavors.
5. Pour in the diced tomatoes (with their juices) and coconut milk. Stir well to combine.
6. Add the mixed vegetables and cooked lentils to the pot. Season with salt and pepper to taste.

7. Simmer the curry over medium-low heat until the vegetables are tender, and the flavors meld together (about 15-20 minutes).

8. Garnish the curry with fresh chopped cilantro before serving.

For the Whole-Grain Naan Bread:

1. In a large bowl, combine whole wheat flour, baking powder, baking soda, and salt.

2. In a separate bowl, mix together yogurt and olive oil. Add the wet ingredients to the dry ingredients, stirring until a dough forms.

3. Knead the dough on a floured surface until it becomes smooth.

4. Divide the dough into small portions and roll each into a ball. Roll out each ball into a flat, oval shape (naan).

5. Optional: For garlic naan, sprinkle minced garlic on the rolled-out naan and press it lightly into the dough.

6. Heat a non-stick skillet over medium-high heat. Cook each naan for 1-2 minutes on each side until it puffs up and develops a golden brown color.

Snack: Mixed nuts (walnuts, almonds, and pistachios)

Ingredients:

- 1 cup raw walnuts
- 1 cup raw almonds
- 1 cup raw pistachios (shelled)
- 1 tablespoon olive oil
- 1 tablespoon honey
- 1 teaspoon ground cinnamon
- 1/2 teaspoon sea salt (adjust to taste)

Instructions:

1. Preheat your oven to 325°F (163°C).
2. In a large mixing bowl, combine walnuts, almonds, and pistachios.
3. In a small bowl, whisk together olive oil, honey, ground cinnamon, and sea salt until well combined.
4. Pour the honey mixture over the mixed nuts and toss until all nuts are evenly coated.
5. Spread the coated nuts in a single layer on a baking sheet lined with parchment paper.
6. Roast the nuts in the preheated oven for 15-20 minutes, stirring halfway through to ensure even roasting. Keep a close eye to prevent burning.

7. Remove the nuts from the oven when they are golden brown and fragrant.

8. Allow the nuts to cool on the baking sheet. They will continue to crisp up as they cool.

9. Once completely cooled, transfer the roasted mixed nuts to an airtight container for storage.

10. Enjoy the roasted mixed nuts as a snack, or use them as a crunchy topping for salads, yogurt, or desserts.

Dinner: Baked cod with quinoa and roasted sweet potatoes

Ingredients:

For Baked Cod:

- 4 cod filets
- 2 tablespoons olive oil
- 2 cloves garlic, minced
- 1 teaspoon paprika
- 1 teaspoon dried oregano
- Salt and pepper to taste
- Lemon wedges for serving

For Quinoa:

- 1 cup quinoa, rinsed
- 2 cups water or vegetable broth

- Salt to taste

For Roasted Sweet Potatoes:

- 2 medium sweet potatoes, peeled and diced
- 2 tablespoons olive oil
- 1 teaspoon smoked paprika
- Salt and pepper to taste

Instructions:

1. Preheat your oven to 400°F (200°C).

2. Marinate the cod filets: In a small bowl, mix together olive oil, minced garlic, paprika, dried oregano, salt, and pepper. Coat each cod filet with this mixture, ensuring they are well-seasoned.

3. Place the marinated cod filets in a baking dish. Bake in the preheated oven for about 15-20 minutes, or until the cod is opaque and flakes easily with a fork.

4. While the cod is baking, prepare the quinoa: In a saucepan, combine rinsed quinoa and water or vegetable broth. Bring to a boil, then reduce heat to low, cover, and simmer for 15-20 minutes or until the quinoa is cooked and water is absorbed. Fluff with a fork and set aside.

5. Roast the sweet potatoes: Toss the diced sweet potatoes with olive oil, smoked paprika, salt, and pepper. Spread them on a baking sheet in a single layer. Roast in the oven for 20-25 minutes or until the sweet potatoes are tender and slightly caramelized.

6. Once everything is ready, assemble the meal: Place a portion of quinoa on each plate, top with a baked cod fillet, and serve alongside the roasted sweet potatoes.

7. Garnish with fresh herbs, if desired, and serve with lemon wedges for a citrusy touch.

8. Enjoy your balanced and flavorful meal of baked cod, quinoa, and roasted sweet potatoes!

Day 5:

Breakfast: Greek yogurt parfait with granola and mixed berries

Ingredients:

- 2 cups Greek yogurt
- 1 cup granola

- 1 cup mixed berries (strawberries, blueberries, raspberries)
- 2 tablespoons honey
- 1 teaspoon vanilla extract
- Mint leaves for garnish (optional)

Instructions:

1. In a bowl, mix Greek yogurt with honey and vanilla extract. Stir until well combined.
2. Wash and prepare the mixed berries. If using strawberries, slice them into bite-sized pieces.
3. Choose serving glasses or bowls for your parfaits.
4. Begin assembling the parfaits by layering a spoonful of Greek yogurt at the bottom of each glass.
5. Add a layer of granola on top of the yogurt. Ensure an even distribution.
6. Place a handful of mixed berries over the granola layer. Be creative with the arrangement for a visually appealing parfait.
7. Repeat the layers until you reach the top of the glass, finishing with a final layer of berries.
8. Drizzle a bit of honey on the top for added sweetness and presentation.

9. Optionally, garnish with fresh mint leaves to enhance the visual appeal and add a hint of freshness.

10. Serve immediately or refrigerate until ready to eat.

Lunch: Spinach and kale salad with grilled chicken, avocado, and citrus vinaigrette

Ingredients:

For the Salad:

- 4 cups baby spinach leaves, washed and dried
- 2 cups kale leaves, stems removed, finely chopped
- 1 pound boneless, skinless chicken breasts, grilled and sliced
- 1 ripe avocado, peeled, pitted, and sliced

For the Citrus Vinaigrette:

- 1/4 cup extra-virgin olive oil
- 2 tablespoons fresh orange juice
- 1 tablespoon fresh lemon juice
- 1 teaspoon Dijon mustard
- 1 clove garlic, minced

- Salt and black pepper to taste

Optional Toppings:

- Cherry tomatoes, halved
- Red onion, thinly sliced
- Toasted nuts (such as almonds or walnuts)

Instructions:

For the Salad:

1. In a large salad bowl, combine the baby spinach and finely chopped kale.
2. Add the grilled and sliced chicken on top of the greens.
3. Arrange sliced avocado over the salad.
4. Optional: Add cherry tomatoes, thinly sliced red onion, or toasted nuts for additional flavor and texture.

For the Citrus Vinaigrette:

1. In a small bowl, whisk together extra-virgin olive oil, fresh orange juice, fresh lemon juice, Dijon mustard, minced garlic, salt, and black pepper.
2. Adjust the seasoning to taste and ensure the vinaigrette is well emulsified.

Assembling the Salad:

1. Drizzle the citrus vinaigrette over the salad.

2. Toss the salad gently to ensure even coating of the dressing.

3. Serve immediately, ensuring each portion has a mix of greens, grilled chicken, avocado, and optional toppings.

4. Enjoy this flavorful and nutritious spinach and kale salad with grilled chicken and citrus vinaigrette!

Snack: Sliced cucumber with hummus

Ingredients:

- 2 medium-sized cucumbers, washed and sliced
- 1 cup hummus (store-bought or homemade)
- 1 tablespoon olive oil
- 1 teaspoon lemon juice
- Salt and pepper to taste
- Optional: Fresh herbs (such as parsley or dill) for garnish

Instructions:

1. Start by washing the cucumbers thoroughly. You can peel them if you prefer, or leave the skin on for added texture and nutrition. Slice the cucumbers into rounds or diagonal slices, depending on your preference.

2. In a small bowl, prepare the dressing by mixing olive oil, lemon juice, salt, and pepper. Adjust the seasoning to taste.

3. Arrange the cucumber slices on a serving platter or individual plates.

4. Spoon dollops of hummus over the cucumber slices. You can spread it evenly or leave it rustic for a more casual presentation.

5. Drizzle the prepared dressing over the cucumber and hummus. Ensure it's evenly distributed.

6. If desired, garnish with fresh herbs like parsley or dill. This adds a burst of flavor and a touch of freshness.

7. Serve immediately as a refreshing appetizer, snack, or a light side dish.

Dinner: Stir-fried tofu with broccoli and brown rice

Ingredients:

- 1 block extra-firm tofu, pressed and cubed
- 2 cups broccoli florets
- 1 cup sliced bell peppers (any color)
- 2 cloves garlic, minced
- 1 tablespoon ginger, grated

- 3 tablespoons soy sauce

- 2 tablespoons hoisin sauce

- 1 tablespoon sesame oil

- 2 tablespoons vegetable oil

- 2 cups cooked brown rice

- Sesame seeds for garnish (optional)

- Green onions, chopped, for garnish (optional)

Instructions:

1. Press the tofu to remove excess water by wrapping it in a clean kitchen towel and placing something heavy on top for about 15-20 minutes. Once pressed, cut the tofu into cubes.

2. Heat 1 tablespoon of vegetable oil in a large pan or wok over medium-high heat. Add the tofu cubes and cook until golden brown on all sides. Remove tofu from the pan and set aside.

3. In the same pan, add another tablespoon of vegetable oil. Stir in the minced garlic and grated ginger, cooking for about 30 seconds until fragrant.

4. Add the broccoli florets and sliced bell peppers to the pan. Stir-fry for 3-4 minutes until the vegetables are slightly tender but still crisp.

5. In a small bowl, whisk together soy sauce, hoisin sauce, and sesame oil. Pour the sauce over the vegetables in the pan.

6. Add the cooked tofu back to the pan, tossing everything together to coat in the sauce. Cook for an additional 2-3 minutes, allowing the tofu and vegetables to absorb the flavors.

7. Serve the stir-fried tofu and vegetables over cooked brown rice.

8. Garnish with sesame seeds and chopped green onions if desired.

Day 6:

Breakfast: Whole-grain toast with avocado and poached eggs

Ingredients:

- 4 slices of whole-grain bread
- 2 ripe avocados
- 4 large eggs
- Vinegar (for poaching eggs)
- Salt and pepper to taste
- Red pepper flakes (optional, for extra heat)

- Fresh chives or parsley, chopped (for garnish)

Instructions:

1. Toast the whole-grain bread slices to your desired level of crispiness.

2. While the bread is toasting, cut the avocados in half, remove the pits, and scoop the flesh into a bowl. Mash the avocado with a fork and season it with salt and pepper. If you like a bit of heat, you can also add red pepper flakes.

3. In a medium-sized skillet, bring water to a gentle simmer. Add a splash of vinegar to the simmering water; this helps the egg whites coagulate more easily when poaching.

4. Crack each egg into a small bowl or ramekin.

5. Create a gentle whirlpool in the simmering water using a spoon, and carefully slide one egg into the center of the whirlpool. Repeat for the remaining eggs.

6. Poach the eggs for about 3-4 minutes for a runny yolk or longer if you prefer a firmer yolk.

7. While the eggs are poaching, spread the mashed avocado evenly onto each slice of toasted whole-grain bread.

8. Using a slotted spoon, carefully lift each poached egg from the water, allowing excess water to drain, and place one egg on top of each avocado-covered toast.

9. Season the poached eggs with a pinch of salt and pepper.

10. Garnish with chopped fresh chives or parsley.

11. Serve immediately, and enjoy your delicious and nutritious whole-grain toast with avocado and poached eggs.

Lunch: Quinoa and black bean bowl with salsa and guacamole

Ingredients:

For Quinoa and Black Bean Bowl:

- 1 cup quinoa, rinsed and drained
- 2 cups water or vegetable broth
- 1 can (15 oz) black beans, drained and rinsed
- 1 cup corn kernels (fresh or frozen)
- 1 red bell pepper, diced
- 1 avocado, sliced
- Fresh cilantro, chopped (for garnish)
- Lime wedges (for serving)

For Salsa:

- 1 cup diced tomatoes
- 1/2 cup diced red onion
- 1/4 cup chopped fresh cilantro
- 1 jalapeño, seeded and finely chopped
- 1 clove garlic, minced
- Salt and pepper to taste

For Guacamole:

- 2 ripe avocados
- 1/4 cup diced red onion
- 1 clove garlic, minced
- 1 tablespoon lime juice
- Salt and pepper to taste

Instructions:

1. In a medium saucepan, combine quinoa and water or vegetable broth. Bring to a boil, then reduce heat to low, cover, and simmer for 15-20 minutes or until quinoa is cooked and water is absorbed. Fluff with a fork.

2. While the quinoa is cooking, prepare the salsa by combining diced tomatoes, red onion, cilantro, jalapeño, garlic, salt, and pepper in a bowl. Mix well and set aside.

3. In another bowl, make the guacamole by mashing ripe avocados and combining them with diced red onion, minced garlic, lime juice, salt, and pepper. Mix until smooth.

4. In a skillet, heat the black beans and corn until warmed through.

5. Assemble the quinoa and black bean bowls by dividing the cooked quinoa among serving bowls. Top with black beans, corn, diced red bell pepper, avocado slices, and a generous spoonful of salsa.

6. Garnish the bowls with chopped cilantro and serve with lime wedges on the side.

7. Optionally, serve with tortilla chips for added crunch.

Snack: Orange slices with a handful of sunflower seeds

Ingredients:

- 4 large navel oranges
- 1/4 cup sunflower seeds
- Honey (optional, for drizzling)
- Mint leaves (optional, for garnish)

Instructions:

1. Peel the oranges and cut them into thin slices or wedges. Remove any seeds.

2. Arrange the orange slices on a serving platter or individual plates.

3. In a dry skillet over medium heat, toast the sunflower seeds for 2-3 minutes, or until they become lightly golden and aromatic. Stir frequently to avoid burning.

4. Sprinkle the toasted sunflower seeds over the orange slices.

5. If desired, drizzle a bit of honey over the orange slices and sunflower seeds for added sweetness. This step is optional, as the natural sweetness of the oranges is usually sufficient.

6. Garnish the dish with fresh mint leaves for a burst of color and added freshness.

7. Serve the orange slices with sunflower seeds immediately as a refreshing and nutritious snack or light dessert.

Dinner: Grilled turkey burgers with a side of roasted vegetables

Ingredients:

For Turkey Burgers:

- 1.5 lbs ground turkey
- 1/4 cup breadcrumbs
- 1/4 cup finely chopped onion
- 2 cloves garlic, minced
- 1 teaspoon dried oregano
- 1 teaspoon dried basil
- Salt and pepper to taste
- 4 whole wheat burger buns

For Roasted Vegetables:

- 2 cups mixed vegetables (such as bell peppers, zucchini, cherry tomatoes)
- 2 tablespoons olive oil
- 1 teaspoon dried thyme
- Salt and pepper to taste

Instructions:

For Turkey Burgers:

1. In a large mixing bowl, combine ground turkey, breadcrumbs, chopped onion, minced garlic, dried oregano, dried basil, salt, and pepper.

2. Mix the ingredients gently but thoroughly. Divide the mixture into four portions and shape them into burger patties.

3. Preheat your grill or grill pan over medium-high heat. Lightly oil the grates to prevent sticking.

4. Place the turkey patties on the grill and cook for about 5-7 minutes per side or until the internal temperature reaches 165°F (74°C).

5. Toast the whole wheat burger buns on the grill for a minute or two until they are lightly browned.

6. Assemble the burgers by placing each turkey patty on a bun. You can add your favorite toppings such as lettuce, tomato, and condiments.

For Roasted Vegetables:

1. Preheat the oven to 400°F (200°C).

2. In a large bowl, toss the mixed vegetables with olive oil, dried thyme, salt, and pepper until well coated.

3. Spread the seasoned vegetables on a baking sheet in a single layer.

4. Roast in the preheated oven for about 20-25 minutes or until the vegetables are tender and slightly caramelized, stirring halfway through.

5. Once roasted, remove the vegetables from the oven and serve alongside the grilled turkey burgers.

Day 7:

Breakfast: Berry and kale smoothie with a touch of ginger

Ingredients:

- 1 cup fresh or frozen mixed berries (such as strawberries, blueberries, raspberries)
- 1 cup kale leaves, stems removed and chopped
- 1 banana, peeled
- 1/2 cup plain Greek yogurt
- 1 tablespoon chia seeds
- 1 teaspoon grated fresh ginger
- 1 cup almond milk (or any milk of your choice)
- Ice cubes (optional)
- Honey or agave syrup (optional, for added sweetness)

Instructions:

1. Place the mixed berries, chopped kale, banana, Greek yogurt, chia seeds, and grated ginger in a blender.

2. Pour in the almond milk and add ice cubes if desired. The ice cubes will give your smoothie a refreshing and frosty texture.

3. Blend the ingredients on high speed until the mixture is smooth and creamy. If the consistency is too thick, you can add more almond milk to reach your desired thickness.

4. Taste the smoothie and, if needed, add honey or agave syrup for additional sweetness. Blend again to combine.

5. Once the smoothie reaches the desired consistency and taste, pour it into glasses.

6. Garnish with extra berries or a sprinkle of chia seeds if you like.

7. Serve immediately and enjoy your nutrient-packed berry and kale smoothie with a touch of ginger.

Lunch: Lentil and vegetable soup with whole-grain crackers

Ingredients:

- 1 cup dry lentils (green or brown), rinsed and drained
- 1 onion, finely chopped
- 2 carrots, diced
- 2 celery stalks, chopped
- 3 cloves garlic, minced
- 1 can (14 oz) diced tomatoes, undrained
- 6 cups vegetable broth
- 1 teaspoon ground cumin
- 1 teaspoon ground coriander
- 1/2 teaspoon smoked paprika
- Salt and pepper to taste
- 2 cups mixed vegetables (e.g., zucchini, bell peppers, spinach)
- 1 cup whole-grain crackers

Instructions:

1. In a large soup pot, combine the rinsed lentils, chopped onion, diced carrots, chopped celery, minced garlic, diced tomatoes (with their juice), and vegetable broth.

2. Add ground cumin, ground coriander, smoked paprika, salt, and pepper to the pot. Stir well to combine all the ingredients.

3. Bring the soup to a boil, then reduce the heat to low, cover, and let it simmer for about 25-30 minutes or until the lentils are tender.

4. Add the mixed vegetables to the pot and continue to simmer for an additional 10-15 minutes, or until the vegetables are cooked to your liking.

5. Adjust the seasoning if needed and let the soup rest for a few minutes to allow the flavors to meld.

6. While the soup is resting, serve it with whole-grain crackers on the side. You can crush some crackers on top of the soup for an extra crunch.

7. Ladle the lentil and vegetable soup into bowls, and enjoy a warm, hearty meal.

Snack: Cottage cheese with pineapple chunks

Ingredients:

- 1 cup cottage cheese

- 1 cup fresh pineapple chunks
- 2 tablespoons honey
- 1/4 cup chopped mint leaves (optional)
- 1/4 cup chopped nuts (such as almonds or walnuts)

Instructions:

1. In a mixing bowl, combine the cottage cheese and fresh pineapple chunks.

2. Drizzle honey over the mixture and gently toss everything together until well combined. Adjust the amount of honey to your desired level of sweetness.

3. If you like a hint of freshness, add chopped mint leaves to the bowl and toss them with the cottage cheese and pineapple.

4. Sprinkle chopped nuts (almonds or walnuts work well) over the mixture for added crunch and flavor.

5. Once all the ingredients are well combined, refrigerate the cottage cheese with pineapple for at least 30 minutes to let the flavors meld.

6. Before serving, give the mixture a final gentle toss. You can garnish with extra mint leaves or nuts for a decorative touch.

7. Serve chilled as a refreshing and nutritious snack or light dessert.

Dinner: Baked salmon with quinoa and steamed green beans

Ingredients:

- 4 salmon filets
- 1 cup quinoa
- 2 cups water or chicken/vegetable broth
- 1 pound green beans, trimmed
- 2 tablespoons olive oil
- 2 cloves garlic, minced
- 1 teaspoon lemon zest
- 2 tablespoons lemon juice
- 1 teaspoon dried oregano
- Salt and pepper to taste
- Fresh parsley for garnish

Instructions:

1. Preheat your oven to 375°F (190°C).
2. Rinse the quinoa under cold water. In a medium saucepan, combine quinoa and water (or broth).

3. Bring to a boil, then reduce heat to low, cover, and simmer for 15-20 minutes or until the liquid is absorbed and quinoa is tender. Fluff with a fork and set aside.

4. Place the salmon filets on a baking sheet lined with parchment paper. Season with salt, pepper, and dried oregano. Drizzle with olive oil and sprinkle minced garlic over the filets. Bake in the preheated oven for 15-20 minutes or until the salmon easily flakes with a fork.

5. While the salmon is baking, steam the green beans. You can use a steamer basket or place them in a microwave-safe dish with a bit of water. Steam until they are tender but still crisp, usually about 5-7 minutes.

6. In a small bowl, whisk together lemon zest, lemon juice, and a bit more olive oil. Season with salt and pepper to taste.

7. Once the salmon is done, assemble the plates by placing a portion of quinoa, a salmon filet, and a serving of steamed green beans. Drizzle the lemon dressing over the top and garnish with fresh parsley.

8. Serve immediately and enjoy your baked salmon with quinoa and steamed green beans!

CHAPTER 3: BREAKFAST OPTIONS

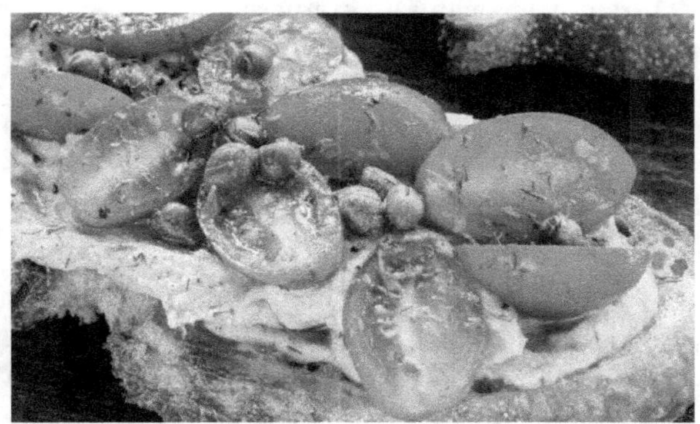

Quinoa Breakfast Bowl

Ingredients:

- 1 cup quinoa, rinsed
- 2 cups water
- 1 cup almond milk (or any milk of your choice)
- 1 tablespoon maple syrup or honey
- 1 teaspoon vanilla extract
- 1/2 teaspoon cinnamon
- Pinch of salt
- Toppings: Fresh berries, sliced banana, nuts, seeds, Greek yogurt

Instructions:

1. Rinse the quinoa thoroughly under cold water to remove its natural bitterness.
2. In a medium saucepan, combine the rinsed quinoa and water. Bring it to a boil over medium-high heat.
3. Once boiling, reduce the heat to low, cover, and simmer for about 15 minutes or until the quinoa is cooked and the water is absorbed.
4. While the quinoa is cooking, prepare the sweetened almond milk. In a separate small saucepan, heat the almond milk over medium heat. Add maple syrup (or honey), vanilla extract, cinnamon, and a pinch of salt. Stir until well combined and heated through.
5. Once the quinoa is cooked, fluff it with a fork and then pour the sweetened almond milk mixture over it. Stir to combine, ensuring the quinoa is well-coated with the sweetened milk.
6. Let the quinoa mixture simmer for an additional 5 minutes, allowing it to absorb the flavors.

7. Remove the saucepan from heat and let it sit, covered, for a few minutes to allow any remaining liquid to be absorbed.

8. Serve the quinoa in bowls and top with your favorite toppings such as fresh berries, sliced banana, nuts, seeds, and a dollop of Greek yogurt.

9. Optionally, drizzle with additional maple syrup or honey for added sweetness.

Turmeric Oatmeal

Ingredients:

- 1 cup rolled oats
- 2 cups water
- 1 cup milk (dairy or plant-based)
- 1 teaspoon ground turmeric
- 1/2 teaspoon ground cinnamon
- 1/4 teaspoon ground ginger
- Pinch of black pepper (enhances turmeric absorption)
- Pinch of salt
- Sweetener to taste (maple syrup, honey, agave syrup)

- Toppings: Sliced banana, chopped nuts, dried fruits, yogurt

Instructions:

1. In a medium-sized saucepan, combine rolled oats, water, and milk.
2. Place the saucepan over medium heat and bring the mixture to a gentle boil, stirring occasionally.
3. Once it starts boiling, reduce the heat to low and add ground turmeric, ground cinnamon, ground ginger, black pepper, and a pinch of salt. Stir well to incorporate the spices evenly into the oatmeal.
4. Simmer the oatmeal on low heat, stirring occasionally, for about 5-7 minutes or until the oats are cooked and the mixture reaches your desired consistency.
5. Add sweetener to taste, such as maple syrup, honey, or agave syrup. Adjust the amount based on your preference for sweetness.
6. Remove the saucepan from heat and let it sit for a minute to allow the flavors to meld.
7. Pour the turmeric oatmeal into bowls and top with sliced banana, chopped nuts, dried fruits, or a dollop of yogurt.

8. Optionally, sprinkle a bit more ground cinnamon on top for added flavor.

9. Serve warm and enjoy your nutritious and golden-hued turmeric oatmeal!

Smoothie Bowl with Greens

Ingredients:

- 1 cup fresh spinach or kale leaves (stems removed)
- 1 ripe banana, peeled and frozen
- 1/2 cup frozen mixed berries (such as strawberries, blueberries, raspberries)
- 1/2 cup plain Greek yogurt or dairy-free yogurt
- 1/2 cup almond milk or any milk of your choice
- 1 tablespoon chia seeds (optional)
- 1 tablespoon nut butter (almond butter, peanut butter, or your choice)
- 1 teaspoon honey or maple syrup (optional, for added sweetness)
- Toppings: Sliced fruits, granola, shredded coconut, nuts, seeds

Instructions:

1. In a blender, combine fresh spinach or kale leaves, frozen banana, frozen mixed berries, Greek yogurt, almond milk, chia seeds (if using), nut butter, and honey or maple syrup (if desired).

2. Blend the ingredients until smooth and creamy. If the mixture is too thick, you can add more almond milk in small increments until you reach your desired consistency.

3. Taste the smoothie and adjust sweetness if necessary by adding more honey or maple syrup. Blend again to combine.

4. Pour the green smoothie into a bowl.

5. Top the smoothie bowl with sliced fruits, granola, shredded coconut, nuts, and seeds. Get creative with the toppings based on your preferences.

6. Optionally, drizzle a bit of honey or nut butter on top for added flavor.

7. Serve the smoothie bowl immediately and enjoy the refreshing and nutrient-packed goodness.

Avocado Toast with Tomato Salsa

Ingredients:

- 2 slices of whole-grain bread
- 1 ripe avocado
- 1 medium-sized tomato, diced
- 1/4 red onion, finely chopped
- 1/4 cup fresh cilantro, chopped
- 1 tablespoon lime juice
- Salt and pepper to taste
- Optional toppings: Poached or fried egg, chili flakes, feta cheese

Instructions:

1. Toast the whole-grain bread slices to your desired level of crispiness.

2. While the bread is toasting, cut the avocado in half, remove the pit, and scoop the flesh into a bowl. Mash the avocado with a fork and season with a pinch of salt and pepper.

3. In a separate bowl, combine diced tomato, finely chopped red onion, chopped cilantro, lime juice, and a pinch of salt. Mix well to create the tomato salsa.

4. Once the bread is toasted, spread the mashed avocado evenly over each slice.

5. Spoon the tomato salsa generously over the avocado-covered bread.

6. Optional: Top each avocado toast with a poached or fried egg for added protein and richness.

7. Sprinkle chili flakes over the top if you like a bit of heat.

8. If desired, crumble feta cheese over the avocado toast for extra flavor.

9. Serve the avocado toast with tomato salsa immediately, and enjoy a delicious and satisfying breakfast or snack!

Chia Seed Pudding

Ingredients:

- 1/4 cup chia seeds
- 1 cup milk (dairy or plant-based, such as almond milk, coconut milk, or soy milk)
- 1 tablespoon honey or maple syrup (adjust to taste)
- 1/2 teaspoon vanilla extract
- Optional toppings: Fresh berries, sliced fruits, nuts, seeds, granola

Instructions:

1. In a bowl, combine chia seeds, milk, honey or maple syrup, and vanilla extract.

2. Whisk the mixture thoroughly to ensure the chia seeds are well distributed and don't clump together.

3. Let the chia seed mixture sit for about 5 minutes, then whisk again to break up any clumps that may have formed.

4. Cover the bowl and refrigerate the chia seed mixture for at least 2 hours or overnight. This allows the chia seeds to absorb the liquid and create a pudding-like consistency.

5. After refrigeration, give the chia seed pudding a good stir to ensure a smooth texture.

6. Taste the pudding and adjust sweetness if needed by adding more honey or maple syrup.

7. Spoon the chia seed pudding into serving glasses or bowls.

8. Top the pudding with your favorite toppings such as fresh berries, sliced fruits, nuts, seeds, or granola.

9. Serve the chia seed pudding chilled and enjoy a nutritious and delicious treat!

Salmon and Cream Cheese Bagel

Ingredients:

- 1 bagel, sliced and toasted
- 4 ounces smoked salmon
- 4 tablespoons cream cheese
- 1 tablespoon capers, drained
- 1/4 red onion, thinly sliced
- Fresh dill, chopped (for garnish)
- Lemon wedges (optional)

Instructions:

1. Toast the bagel slices to your liking. You can use a toaster or an oven for this step.
2. Once the bagel slices are toasted, spread a generous layer of cream cheese on each half of the bagel.
3. Lay slices of smoked salmon on top of the cream cheese, ensuring an even distribution.
4. Sprinkle capers over the smoked salmon. Capers add a tangy and salty flavor that complements the richness of the salmon.
5. Add thinly sliced red onion on top for a bit of crunch and a touch of sweetness.

6. Garnish the salmon and cream cheese bagel with fresh chopped dill. Dill pairs well with both salmon and cream cheese, adding a burst of freshness.

7. Optionally, squeeze lemon wedges over the top for a citrusy kick. This step is based on personal preference.

8. Bring the two halves of the bagel together to form a sandwich.

9. Serve the salmon and cream cheese bagel immediately and enjoy this classic and flavorful combination!

Greek Yogurt Parfait

Ingredients:

- 1 cup Greek yogurt
- 2 tablespoons honey or maple syrup
- 1/2 teaspoon vanilla extract
- 1/2 cup granola
- 1 cup mixed berries (strawberries, blueberries, raspberries)
- 1 tablespoon chopped nuts (such as almonds or walnuts)
- Optional: Drizzle of honey for serving

Instructions:

1. In a bowl, combine Greek yogurt, honey or maple syrup, and vanilla extract. Mix well until the sweetener is evenly distributed throughout the yogurt.

2. Choose serving glasses or bowls for assembling the parfaits.

3. Spoon a layer of the sweetened Greek yogurt into the bottom of each glass or bowl.

4. Add a layer of granola on top of the yogurt. Ensure an even distribution for a balanced bite.

5. Follow with a layer of mixed berries. You can use fresh or thawed frozen berries depending on your preference and availability.

6. Repeat the layers until you reach the top of the glass or bowl, finishing with a final dollop of Greek yogurt.

7. Top the parfait with chopped nuts for added crunch and nutritional value.

8. Optionally, drizzle a bit of honey over the top for extra sweetness.

9. Repeat the assembly process for additional parfaits.

10. Serve the Greek yogurt parfait immediately, or refrigerate until ready to enjoy. The layers can meld together for an even more delicious experience.

Sweet Potato Hash

Ingredients:

- 2 medium-sized sweet potatoes, peeled and diced into small cubes
- 1 bell pepper, diced
- 1 onion, finely chopped
- 2 cloves garlic, minced
- 2 tablespoons olive oil
- 1 teaspoon smoked paprika
- 1/2 teaspoon cumin
- 1/2 teaspoon chili powder (adjust to taste)
- Salt and pepper to taste
- Fresh parsley or cilantro, chopped (for garnish)
- Optional toppings: Fried or poached eggs, avocado slices, hot sauce

Instructions:

1. In a large skillet, heat olive oil over medium heat.

2. Add chopped onions and minced garlic to the skillet. Sauté until the onions become translucent and the garlic is fragrant.

3. Add diced sweet potatoes to the skillet. Spread them out in an even layer to ensure even cooking.

4. Season the sweet potatoes with smoked paprika, cumin, chili powder, salt, and pepper. Stir to coat the sweet potatoes evenly with the spices.

5. Cook the sweet potatoes, stirring occasionally, for about 15-20 minutes or until they are tender and golden brown.

6. Add diced bell pepper to the skillet and cook for an additional 5 minutes, allowing the peppers to soften.

7. Taste the sweet potato hash and adjust the seasoning if necessary.

8. If desired, make wells in the hash and crack eggs into them. Cover the skillet and cook until the eggs are cooked to your liking.

9. Garnish the sweet potato hash with chopped fresh parsley or cilantro.

10. Serve the sweet potato hash hot, with optional toppings such as avocado slices or a drizzle of hot sauce.

Berry and Walnut Pancakes

Ingredients:

- 1 cup all-purpose flour
- 2 tablespoons sugar
- 1 teaspoon baking powder
- 1/2 teaspoon baking soda
- 1/4 teaspoon salt
- 1 cup buttermilk
- 1 large egg
- 2 tablespoons unsalted butter, melted
- 1 teaspoon vanilla extract
- 1/2 cup fresh berries (such as blueberries, raspberries, or sliced strawberries)
- 1/4 cup chopped walnuts
- Maple syrup (for serving)

Instructions:

1. In a large mixing bowl, whisk together the flour, sugar, baking powder, baking soda, and salt.

2. In a separate bowl, whisk together the buttermilk, egg, melted butter, and vanilla extract.

3. Pour the wet ingredients into the dry ingredients and gently stir until just combined. Be careful not to overmix; a few lumps are okay.

4. Gently fold in the fresh berries and chopped walnuts into the pancake batter.

5. Heat a griddle or non-stick skillet over medium heat. Lightly grease with butter or cooking spray.

6. Pour 1/4 cup portions of batter onto the griddle for each pancake.

7. Cook until bubbles form on the surface of the pancake, then flip and cook until the other side is golden brown.

8. Continue cooking the remaining batter, adjusting the heat if necessary to prevent burning.

9. Once all the pancakes are cooked, stack them on a plate.

10. Serve the berry and walnut pancakes warm, drizzled with maple syrup.

Cottage Cheese and Pineapple Bowl

Ingredients:

- 1 cup cottage cheese
- 1 cup fresh pineapple chunks
- 1/4 cup granola
- 1 tablespoon honey or maple syrup
- 2 tablespoons shredded coconut
- 1 tablespoon chopped mint (optional, for garnish)

Instructions:

1. In a bowl, spoon the cottage cheese as the base for your bowl.
2. Add fresh pineapple chunks on top of the cottage cheese. Ensure an even distribution for a balanced bite.
3. Sprinkle granola over the cottage cheese and pineapple. This adds a delightful crunch and additional flavor.
4. Drizzle honey or maple syrup over the bowl for sweetness. Adjust the amount based on your preference.
5. Sprinkle shredded coconut over the top for a tropical touch.

6. Optional: Garnish with chopped mint for a burst of freshness.

7. Mix the ingredients gently in the bowl to combine the flavors.

8. Serve the cottage cheese and pineapple bowl immediately, and enjoy this refreshing and protein-packed treat!

Mushroom and Spinach Omelet

Ingredients:

- 3 large eggs
- 1/2 cup fresh spinach, chopped
- 1/2 cup mushrooms, sliced
- 1/4 cup onion, finely chopped
- 1/4 cup shredded cheese (such as cheddar or feta)
- 1 tablespoon butter or olive oil
- Salt and pepper to taste
- Fresh herbs (optional, for garnish)

Instructions:

1. In a bowl, whisk the eggs until well beaten. Season with a pinch of salt and pepper.

2. Heat butter or olive oil in a non-stick skillet over medium heat.

3. Add chopped onions and sliced mushrooms to the skillet. Sauté until the mushrooms are tender and the onions are translucent.

4. Add chopped spinach to the skillet and cook until wilted. This should take only a minute or two.

5. Pour the beaten eggs over the vegetables in the skillet. Allow the eggs to set slightly at the edges.

6. Using a spatula, gently lift the edges of the omelet, tilting the skillet to let the uncooked egg flow to the edges.

7. Once the edges are set but the top is still slightly runny, sprinkle shredded cheese over one half of the omelet.

8. Carefully fold the other half of the omelet over the cheese-covered half, creating a half-moon shape.

9. Cook for an additional minute or until the cheese is melted and the omelet is cooked to your liking.

10. Slide the mushroom and spinach omelet onto a plate. Garnish with fresh herbs if desired.

11. Serve the omelet hot and enjoy a delicious and nutritious breakfast or brunch!

Coconut Almond Breakfast Bars

Ingredients:

- 1 1/2 cups rolled oats
- 1/2 cup unsweetened shredded coconut
- 1/2 cup almonds, chopped
- 1/4 cup honey or maple syrup
- 1/4 cup almond butter
- 1/4 cup coconut oil, melted
- 1 teaspoon vanilla extract
- 1/4 teaspoon salt

Instructions:

1. Preheat your oven to 350°F (175°C). Grease or line an 8x8-inch baking pan with parchment paper.

2. In a large mixing bowl, combine rolled oats, shredded coconut, and chopped almonds.

3. In a small saucepan, heat honey or maple syrup, almond butter, melted coconut oil, vanilla extract, and salt over low heat. Stir until the mixture is well combined and smooth.

4. Pour the wet ingredients over the dry ingredients in the large mixing bowl. Stir until all the ingredients are evenly coated.

5. Transfer the mixture into the prepared baking pan. Use a spatula to press the mixture down firmly and create an even layer.

6. Bake in the preheated oven for about 15-20 minutes or until the edges are golden brown.

7. Remove the pan from the oven and let it cool completely before cutting into bars.

8. Once cooled, cut the mixture into bars or squares.

9. Store the coconut almond breakfast bars in an airtight container. They can be kept at room temperature for a few days or refrigerated for longer shelf life.

10. Enjoy these homemade bars as a delicious and wholesome breakfast or snack!

Veggie Frittata

Ingredients:

- 8 large eggs
- 1/2 cup milk
- Salt and pepper to taste

- 2 tablespoons olive oil
- 1 small onion, finely chopped
- 2 bell peppers (any color), diced
- 1 zucchini, diced
- 1 cup cherry tomatoes, halved
- 1 cup spinach, chopped
- 1/2 cup feta cheese, crumbled (optional)
- Fresh herbs (such as parsley or chives) for garnish

Instructions:

1. Preheat your oven to 375°F (190°C).
2. In a bowl, whisk together the eggs, milk, salt, and pepper until well combined. Set aside.
3. Heat olive oil in an oven-safe skillet over medium heat. Add the chopped onion and sauté until softened, about 2-3 minutes.
4. Add the diced bell peppers and zucchini to the skillet. Cook for another 5-7 minutes or until the vegetables are tender.
5. Stir in the cherry tomatoes and chopped spinach. Cook for an additional 2-3 minutes until the spinach wilts.

6. Pour the egg mixture over the sautéed vegetables in the skillet. Allow the eggs to set around the edges.

7. Sprinkle crumbled feta cheese over the top if using. Transfer the skillet to the preheated oven.

8. Bake for 15-20 minutes or until the frittata is set in the center and has a golden brown color on top.

9. Remove the skillet from the oven (be cautious as the handle will be hot). Let it cool for a few minutes.

10. Garnish the veggie frittata with fresh herbs, slice into wedges, and serve. Enjoy your delicious and nutritious veggie frittata!

Orange Ginger Carrot Smoothie

Ingredients:

- 2 cups carrots, peeled and chopped
- 1 orange, peeled and segmented
- 1-inch piece of fresh ginger, peeled and grated
- 1 banana
- 1 cup plain Greek yogurt
- 1-2 tablespoons honey (adjust to taste)
- 1 cup ice cubes

- 1/2 cup water or orange juice (adjust for desired consistency)

Instructions:

1. Start by preparing the ingredients. Peel and chop the carrots, peel and segment the orange, and peel and grate the fresh ginger.
2. In a blender, combine the chopped carrots, orange segments, grated ginger, banana, Greek yogurt, honey, and ice cubes.
3. Add water or orange juice to the blender to help with blending. Start with 1/2 cup and adjust based on your desired smoothie consistency.
4. Blend the ingredients on high speed until the mixture is smooth and creamy. Pause and scrape down the sides of the blender if needed.
5. Taste the smoothie and adjust the sweetness by adding more honey if necessary.
6. Once the smoothie reaches your desired consistency and taste, pour it into glasses.
7. Garnish with a slice of orange or a sprinkle of grated ginger if you like.
8. Serve immediately and enjoy your refreshing and nutritious Orange Ginger Carrot Smoothie!

CHAPTER 4: LUNCH RECIPES

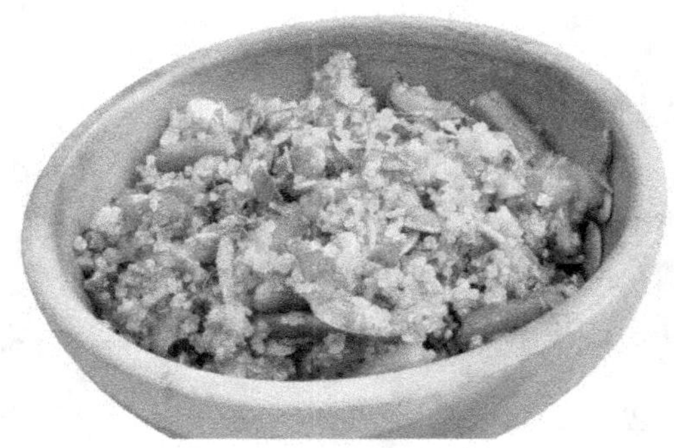

Salmon Salad with Mixed Greens

Ingredients:

- 1 lb salmon filets
- Salt and black pepper to taste
- 2 tablespoons olive oil
- 1 teaspoon lemon zest
- 2 tablespoons lemon juice
- 1 tablespoon Dijon mustard
- 1 clove garlic, minced
- 4 cups mixed salad greens (e.g., arugula, spinach, romaine)
- 1 cup cherry tomatoes, halved
- 1 cucumber, sliced

- 1/2 red onion, thinly sliced

- 1/4 cup Kalamata olives, pitted and halved

- 1/4 cup feta cheese, crumbled (optional)

- 2 tablespoons fresh dill, chopped

- Lemon wedges for serving

Instructions:

1. Preheat the oven to 400°F (200°C).

2. Season the salmon filets with salt and black pepper. Place them on a baking sheet lined with parchment paper.

3. In a small bowl, mix together olive oil, lemon zest, lemon juice, Dijon mustard, and minced garlic. Brush this mixture over the salmon filets.

4. Bake the salmon in the preheated oven for 12-15 minutes or until it flakes easily with a fork.

5. While the salmon is baking, prepare the salad. In a large bowl, combine the mixed salad greens, cherry tomatoes, cucumber, red onion, and Kalamata olives.

6. Once the salmon is done, let it cool slightly, then break it into large flakes with a fork.

7. Add the salmon flakes to the salad.

8. If desired, sprinkle crumbled feta cheese over the salad.

9. Drizzle the remaining lemon-mustard dressing over the salad and toss gently to combine.

10. Garnish the salad with fresh dill and serve with lemon wedges on the side.

11. Enjoy your Salmon Salad with Mixed Greens as a healthy and flavorful meal!

Quinoa and Vegetable Stir-Fry

Ingredients:

- 1 cup quinoa, rinsed and drained
- 2 cups water
- 2 tablespoons soy sauce
- 1 tablespoon sesame oil
- 1 tablespoon rice vinegar
- 1 tablespoon honey
- 1 tablespoon ginger, minced
- 2 cloves garlic, minced
- 2 tablespoons vegetable oil
- 1 medium carrot, julienned
- 1 red bell pepper, thinly sliced
- 1 yellow bell pepper, thinly sliced
- 1 cup broccoli florets
- 1 cup snap peas, ends trimmed
- 1 cup mushrooms, sliced

- 2 green onions, sliced

- Sesame seeds for garnish (optional)

Instructions:

1. In a medium saucepan, combine quinoa and water. Bring to a boil, then reduce heat to low, cover, and simmer for 15 minutes or until the quinoa is cooked and water is absorbed. Remove from heat and let it sit, covered, for 5 minutes. Fluff with a fork.

2. In a small bowl, whisk together soy sauce, sesame oil, rice vinegar, honey, minced ginger, and minced garlic to create the stir-fry sauce. Set aside.

3. Heat vegetable oil in a large wok or skillet over medium-high heat.

4. Add julienned carrots, sliced bell peppers, broccoli florets, snap peas, and mushrooms to the wok. Stir-fry for 4-5 minutes or until the vegetables are tender-crisp.

5. Push the vegetables to one side of the wok and add the cooked quinoa to the empty space. Pour the stir-fry sauce over the quinoa and toss to coat.

6. Gradually mix the quinoa with the vegetables, ensuring an even distribution of the sauce.

7. Stir in sliced green onions and cook for an additional 1-2 minutes.

8. Taste and adjust the seasoning if needed.

9. Serve the quinoa and vegetable stir-fry hot, garnished with sesame seeds if desired.

10. Enjoy this nutritious and delicious Quinoa and Vegetable Stir-Fry as a satisfying meal!

Lentil Soup with Spinach

Ingredients:

- 1 cup dried green or brown lentils, rinsed and drained
- 1 large onion, finely chopped
- 2 carrots, peeled and diced
- 2 celery stalks, diced
- 3 cloves garlic, minced
- 1 teaspoon ground cumin
- 1 teaspoon ground coriander
- 1/2 teaspoon smoked paprika
- 1/4 teaspoon cayenne pepper (optional, for heat)
- 6 cups vegetable broth
- 1 can (14 oz) diced tomatoes, undrained

- 2 cups fresh spinach, chopped
- 2 tablespoons olive oil
- Salt and black pepper to taste
- Lemon wedges for serving (optional)

Instructions:

1. In a large soup pot, heat olive oil over medium heat. Add chopped onions, carrots, and celery. Sauté for 5-7 minutes or until the vegetables are softened.

2. Add minced garlic, ground cumin, ground coriander, smoked paprika, and cayenne pepper (if using). Sauté for an additional 1-2 minutes until the spices are fragrant.

3. Pour in the vegetable broth, add the rinsed lentils, and bring the mixture to a boil. Reduce the heat, cover, and simmer for about 20-25 minutes or until the lentils are tender.

4. Add the diced tomatoes (with their juice) to the pot. Continue to simmer for an additional 10 minutes.

5. Stir in the chopped fresh spinach and cook until wilted, about 2-3 minutes.

6. Season the lentil soup with salt and black pepper to taste. Adjust the seasoning as needed.

7. Ladle the soup into bowls and serve hot. Optionally, squeeze a lemon wedge over each bowl before eating.

8. Enjoy your comforting and nutritious Lentil Soup with Spinach!

Mushroom and Brown Rice Risotto

Ingredients:

- 1 cup brown rice
- 4 cups vegetable broth
- 2 tablespoons olive oil
- 1 onion, finely chopped
- 2 cloves garlic, minced
- 8 oz mushrooms, sliced (e.g., cremini, shiitake, or a mix)
- 1 cup Arborio rice
- 1/2 cup dry white wine (optional)
- 1 teaspoon thyme, chopped
- 1/2 cup Parmesan cheese, grated
- Salt and black pepper to taste
- Fresh parsley for garnish

Instructions:

1. In a medium saucepan, bring the vegetable broth to a simmer. Keep it warm over low heat.

2. Rinse the brown rice under cold water. In a separate pot, cook the brown rice according to package instructions. This might take around 45-50 minutes. Once cooked, drain any excess water and set aside.

3. In a large skillet or wide saucepan, heat olive oil over medium heat. Add the chopped onion and sauté for 3-4 minutes until softened.

4. Add minced garlic to the skillet and sauté for an additional 1-2 minutes until fragrant.

5. Add the sliced mushrooms to the skillet and cook for 5-7 minutes until they release their moisture and become golden brown.

6. Stir in Arborio rice, ensuring it's well coated with the oil and mixed with the vegetables. Toast the rice for about 2 minutes.

7. If using, pour in the white wine and stir until most of the liquid is absorbed.

8. Begin adding the warm vegetable broth one ladle at a time, stirring frequently. Allow the liquid to be absorbed before adding the next ladle. Continue this process until the Arborio rice is creamy and cooked al dente. This usually takes about 18-20 minutes.

9. Add the cooked brown rice to the skillet, stirring to combine.

10. Stir in chopped thyme and grated Parmesan cheese. Season the risotto with salt and black pepper to taste.

11. Remove the skillet from heat. Garnish the mushroom and brown rice risotto with fresh parsley.

12. Serve immediately, and enjoy your flavorful and creamy Mushroom and Brown Rice Risotto!

Grilled Chicken and Veggie Skewers

Ingredients:

- 1.5 lbs boneless, skinless chicken breasts, cut into cubes
- 1 zucchini, sliced into rounds
- 1 red bell pepper, cut into chunks
- 1 yellow bell pepper, cut into chunks
- 1 red onion, cut into chunks
- Cherry tomatoes
- 2 tablespoons olive oil
- 2 tablespoons balsamic vinegar
- 2 cloves garlic, minced
- 1 teaspoon dried oregano

- 1 teaspoon dried thyme
- Salt and black pepper to taste
- Wooden or metal skewers

Instructions:

1. If using wooden skewers, soak them in water for at least 30 minutes to prevent burning during grilling.
2. In a bowl, mix olive oil, balsamic vinegar, minced garlic, dried oregano, dried thyme, salt, and black pepper to create the marinade.
3. Place the chicken cubes in a separate bowl and coat them with half of the marinade. Allow the chicken to marinate for at least 30 minutes.
4. Preheat your grill to medium-high heat.
5. Thread the marinated chicken, zucchini rounds, bell pepper chunks, red onion chunks, and cherry tomatoes onto the skewers, alternating the ingredients.
6. Brush the skewers with the remaining marinade.
7. Place the skewers on the preheated grill. Grill for 10-12 minutes, turning occasionally, until the chicken is cooked through and the vegetables are charred and tender.

8. Check for doneness by cutting into a piece of chicken to ensure it's no longer pink inside.

9. Remove the skewers from the grill and let them rest for a couple of minutes.

10. Serve the grilled chicken and veggie skewers hot. You can accompany them with your favorite dipping sauce or a side of rice.

11. Enjoy these delicious and flavorful Grilled Chicken and Veggie Skewers!

Sweet Potato and Black Bean Salad

Ingredients:

- 2 medium sweet potatoes, peeled and diced
- 1 can (15 oz) black beans, drained and rinsed
- 1 cup corn kernels (fresh, frozen, or canned)
- 1 red bell pepper, diced
- 1/2 red onion, finely chopped
- 1/4 cup fresh cilantro, chopped
- 1 avocado, diced
- Juice of 2 limes
- 3 tablespoons olive oil
- 1 teaspoon ground cumin
- 1 teaspoon chili powder
- Salt and black pepper to taste

Instructions:

1. Preheat the oven to 400°F (200°C).

2. Place the diced sweet potatoes on a baking sheet. Drizzle with olive oil, sprinkle with salt and pepper, and toss to coat evenly.

3. Roast the sweet potatoes in the preheated oven for 20-25 minutes or until they are tender and slightly caramelized. Stir halfway through the cooking time.

4. While the sweet potatoes are roasting, prepare the dressing. In a small bowl, whisk together lime juice, olive oil, ground cumin, chili powder, salt, and black pepper. Set aside.

5. In a large mixing bowl, combine the roasted sweet potatoes, black beans, corn, diced red bell pepper, chopped red onion, and fresh cilantro.

6. Pour the prepared dressing over the salad ingredients and toss gently to combine.

7. Add diced avocado to the salad and toss again.

8. Taste the salad and adjust the seasoning if needed.

9. Chill the Sweet Potato and Black Bean Salad in the refrigerator for at least 30 minutes to allow the flavors to meld.

10. Before serving, give the salad a final toss and garnish with extra cilantro if desired.

11. Serve chilled and enjoy this vibrant and nutritious Sweet Potato and Black Bean Salad!

Spinach and Berry Salad with Grilled Chicken

Ingredients:

For the Grilled Chicken:

- 1.5 lbs boneless, skinless chicken breasts
- 2 tablespoons olive oil
- 1 teaspoon dried thyme
- 1 teaspoon dried rosemary
- Salt and black pepper to taste

For the Salad:

- 6 cups fresh baby spinach leaves, washed and dried
- 1 cup strawberries, hulled and sliced
- 1 cup blueberries
- 1/2 cup raspberries
- 1/2 cup crumbled feta cheese
- 1/4 cup sliced almonds, toasted

For the Balsamic Vinaigrette:

- 1/4 cup balsamic vinegar

- 1/2 cup extra-virgin olive oil
- 1 tablespoon Dijon mustard
- 1 clove garlic, minced
- 1 teaspoon honey
- Salt and black pepper to taste

Instructions:

For the Grilled Chicken:

1. Preheat your grill to medium-high heat.
2. In a small bowl, mix olive oil, dried thyme, dried rosemary, salt, and black pepper to create a marinade.
3. Coat the chicken breasts with the marinade, ensuring they are well covered.
4. Grill the chicken for 6-8 minutes per side or until the internal temperature reaches 165°F (74°C) and the chicken is no longer pink in the center.
5. Remove the chicken from the grill, let it rest for a few minutes, then slice it into thin strips.

For the Salad:

1. In a large salad bowl, combine fresh baby spinach, sliced strawberries, blueberries, raspberries, crumbled feta cheese, and toasted sliced almonds.

For the Balsamic Vinaigrette:

1. In a small bowl, whisk together balsamic vinegar, extra-virgin olive oil, Dijon mustard, minced garlic, honey, salt, and black pepper.
2. Drizzle the balsamic vinaigrette over the salad and toss gently to coat the ingredients evenly.
3. Top the salad with the grilled chicken strips.
4. Serve immediately, and enjoy your delicious and nutritious Spinach and Berry Salad with Grilled Chicken!

Tomato Basil Quinoa Bowl

Ingredients:

- 1 cup quinoa, rinsed and drained
- 2 cups water or vegetable broth
- 2 tablespoons olive oil
- 4 cloves garlic, minced
- 1 can (14 oz) diced tomatoes, undrained
- 1/2 cup fresh basil, chopped
- Salt and black pepper to taste
- Red pepper flakes (optional, for added heat)
- 1/4 cup grated Parmesan cheese (optional, for garnish)

Instructions:

1. In a medium saucepan, combine quinoa and water or vegetable broth. Bring to a boil, then reduce heat to low, cover, and simmer for 15-20 minutes or until the quinoa is cooked and water is absorbed. Fluff with a fork.

2. While the quinoa is cooking, heat olive oil in a large skillet over medium heat.

3. Add minced garlic to the skillet and sauté for 1-2 minutes until fragrant.

4. Pour in the can of diced tomatoes with their juice. Cook for 5-7 minutes, allowing the tomatoes to break down and release their flavors.

5. Stir in chopped fresh basil and season the tomato mixture with salt, black pepper, and red pepper flakes (if using). Simmer for an additional 2-3 minutes.

6. Once the quinoa is cooked, add it to the skillet with the tomato and basil mixture. Stir well to combine.

7. Taste and adjust the seasoning if needed.

8. If desired, sprinkle grated Parmesan cheese over the tomato basil quinoa bowl.

9. Serve hot, and enjoy this flavorful and simple Tomato Basil Quinoa Bowl!

Chickpea and Vegetable Curry

Ingredients:

- 2 tablespoons vegetable oil
- 1 large onion, finely chopped
- 3 cloves garlic, minced
- 1 tablespoon ginger, grated
- 1 tablespoon curry powder
- 1 teaspoon ground cumin
- 1 teaspoon ground coriander
- 1/2 teaspoon turmeric
- 1/4 teaspoon cayenne pepper (adjust to taste)
- 1 can (14 oz) diced tomatoes
- 1 can (14 oz) chickpeas, drained and rinsed
- 1 medium cauliflower, cut into florets
- 2 medium carrots, peeled and sliced
- 1 can (14 oz) coconut milk
- 1 cup vegetable broth
- Salt and black pepper to taste
- Fresh cilantro for garnish
- Cooked rice or naan for serving

Instructions:

1. In a large pot or Dutch oven, heat vegetable oil over medium heat.

2. Add chopped onion, minced garlic, and grated ginger. Sauté for 3-4 minutes until the onions are soft and translucent.

3. Add curry powder, ground cumin, ground coriander, turmeric, and cayenne pepper to the pot. Stir well to coat the onions in the spices and cook for an additional 2 minutes.

4. Pour in the diced tomatoes and cook for 5 minutes, allowing the tomatoes to break down.

5. Add drained chickpeas, cauliflower florets, and sliced carrots to the pot. Stir to combine with the tomato mixture.

6. Pour in the coconut milk and vegetable broth. Season the curry with salt and black pepper to taste. Stir well.

7. Bring the curry to a simmer, then reduce the heat to low, cover, and let it cook for 20-25 minutes or until the vegetables are tender.

8. Taste and adjust the seasoning if necessary.

9. Serve the chickpea and vegetable curry over cooked rice or with naan.

10. Garnish with fresh cilantro before serving.

11. Enjoy your hearty and flavorful Chickpea and Vegetable Curry!

Baked Cod with Lemon and Herbs

Ingredients:

- 4 cod filets (about 6 ounces each)
- 2 tablespoons olive oil
- 2 tablespoons fresh lemon juice
- Zest of 1 lemon
- 2 cloves garlic, minced
- 1 teaspoon dried oregano
- 1 teaspoon dried thyme
- Salt and black pepper to taste
- Fresh parsley for garnish
- Lemon wedges for serving

Instructions:

1. Preheat your oven to 400°F (200°C).

2. Pat the cod filets dry with paper towels and place them in a baking dish.

3. In a small bowl, whisk together olive oil, fresh lemon juice, lemon zest, minced garlic, dried oregano, dried thyme, salt, and black pepper to create the marinade.

4. Pour the marinade over the cod filets, ensuring they are well coated. Allow the fish to marinate for at least 15-20 minutes.

5. Bake the cod in the preheated oven for 15-18 minutes or until the fish flakes easily with a fork and is opaque throughout.

6. While the cod is baking, you can baste it with the marinade halfway through cooking.

7. Once the cod is done, remove it from the oven and sprinkle with fresh parsley.

8. Serve the baked cod hot, garnished with lemon wedges on the side.

9. Enjoy your light and flavorful Baked Cod with Lemon and Herbs!

Broccoli and Almond Stir-Fry

Ingredients:

- 1 lb broccoli florets
- 2 tablespoons vegetable oil
- 3 cloves garlic, minced
- 1 teaspoon fresh ginger, grated
- 1/4 cup soy sauce
- 2 tablespoons oyster sauce
- 1 tablespoon rice vinegar

- 1 tablespoon honey
- 1 tablespoon cornstarch (optional, for thickening)
- 1/2 cup almonds, sliced and toasted
- Sesame seeds for garnish (optional)
- Cooked rice for serving

Instructions:

1. Steam the broccoli florets for about 3-4 minutes or until they are crisp-tender. Alternatively, blanch them in boiling water for 2-3 minutes. Drain and set aside.

2. In a small bowl, whisk together soy sauce, oyster sauce, rice vinegar, honey, and cornstarch (if using). Set aside.

3. Heat vegetable oil in a large wok or skillet over medium-high heat.

4. Add minced garlic and grated ginger to the wok. Sauté for 1-2 minutes until fragrant.

5. Add the steamed broccoli to the wok and stir-fry for 2-3 minutes, allowing the broccoli to get well-coated with the garlic and ginger.

6. Pour the sauce over the broccoli and toss to combine. Cook for an additional 2-3 minutes until the sauce thickens slightly.

7. Stir in the toasted sliced almonds and cook for another 1-2 minutes.

8. Taste the stir-fry and adjust the seasoning if needed.

9. Remove the broccoli and almond stir-fry from heat.

10. Serve hot over cooked rice.

11. Garnish with sesame seeds if desired.

12. Enjoy your delicious and crunchy Broccoli and Almond Stir-Fry!

Turkey and Vegetable Wrap

Ingredients:

- 1 lb ground turkey
- 1 tablespoon olive oil
- 1 small onion, finely chopped
- 2 cloves garlic, minced
- 1 teaspoon ground cumin
- 1 teaspoon chili powder
- 1/2 teaspoon paprika
- Salt and black pepper to taste
- 1 cup black beans, drained and rinsed
- 1 cup corn kernels (fresh, frozen, or canned)
- 1 cup cherry tomatoes, halved

- 1 cup lettuce, shredded
- 1 avocado, sliced
- 1/2 cup shredded cheddar cheese
- 4 large whole wheat or spinach tortillas
- Sour cream or Greek yogurt for serving (optional)

Instructions:

1. In a large skillet, heat olive oil over medium heat.
2. Add chopped onion and sauté for 3-4 minutes until softened.
3. Add minced garlic to the skillet and sauté for an additional 1-2 minutes until fragrant.
4. Add ground turkey to the skillet, breaking it apart with a spoon. Cook until the turkey is browned and cooked through.
5. Season the turkey with ground cumin, chili powder, paprika, salt, and black pepper. Mix well to evenly distribute the spices.
6. Stir in black beans and corn, cooking for another 2-3 minutes until heated through.
7. Remove the skillet from heat and set aside.
8. Warm the tortillas in a dry skillet or microwave for about 10 seconds to make them more pliable.

9. Assemble the wraps: Spoon the turkey and vegetable mixture onto the center of each tortilla.

10. Top with halved cherry tomatoes, shredded lettuce, sliced avocado, and shredded cheddar cheese.

11. Fold in the sides of the tortilla and then roll it up tightly to create a wrap.

12. Serve the turkey and vegetable wraps immediately, optionally with a side of sour cream or Greek yogurt.

13. Enjoy your tasty and satisfying Turkey and Vegetable Wrap!

Cauliflower and Chickpea Buddha Bowl

Ingredients:

For the Roasted Cauliflower:

- 1 head cauliflower, cut into florets
- 2 tablespoons olive oil
- 1 teaspoon ground cumin
- 1 teaspoon smoked paprika
- Salt and black pepper to taste

For the Chickpeas:

- 1 can (14 oz) chickpeas, drained and rinsed
- 1 tablespoon olive oil
- 1 teaspoon ground cumin
- 1 teaspoon ground coriander
- 1/2 teaspoon garlic powder
- Salt and black pepper to taste

For the Quinoa:

- 1 cup quinoa, rinsed and drained
- 2 cups water or vegetable broth

For the Bowl:

- 4 cups mixed greens (e.g., spinach, kale, arugula)
- 1 avocado, sliced
- 1 cup cherry tomatoes, halved
- 1/4 cup hummus
- Lemon wedges for serving

Instructions:

For the Roasted Cauliflower:

1. Preheat the oven to 425°F (220°C).
2. In a large bowl, toss cauliflower florets with olive oil, ground cumin, smoked paprika, salt, and black pepper until evenly coated.

3. Spread the cauliflower on a baking sheet lined with parchment paper.

4. Roast in the preheated oven for 25-30 minutes or until the cauliflower is golden brown and tender, stirring halfway through.

For the Chickpeas:

1. In a bowl, toss chickpeas with olive oil, ground cumin, ground coriander, garlic powder, salt, and black pepper.

2. Spread the chickpeas on a baking sheet lined with parchment paper.

3. Roast in the oven at 425°F (220°C) for 20-25 minutes or until crispy, shaking the pan occasionally for even cooking.

For the Quinoa:

1. In a medium saucepan, combine quinoa and water or vegetable broth. Bring to a boil, then reduce heat to low, cover, and simmer for 15-20 minutes or until the quinoa is cooked and water is absorbed. Fluff with a fork.

For Assembling the Bowl:

1. Divide the cooked quinoa among four bowls.

2. Top each bowl with roasted cauliflower, roasted chickpeas, mixed greens, sliced avocado, and halved cherry tomatoes.

3. Drizzle hummus over the top of each bowl.

4. Serve the Cauliflower and Chickpea Buddha Bowls with lemon wedges on the side.

5. Enjoy this nutritious and satisfying bowl!

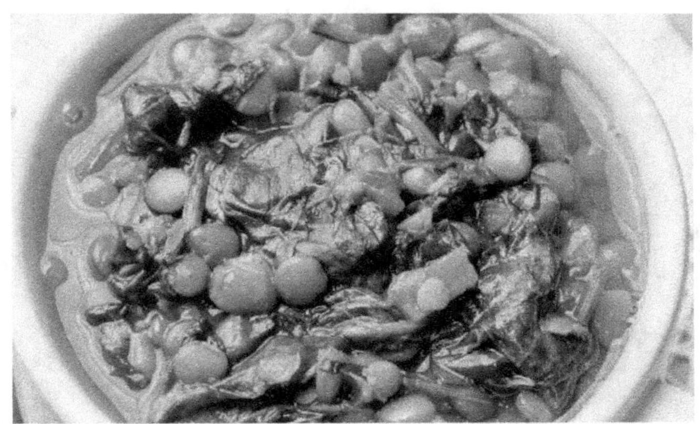

"I embrace the power of
nutritious ingredients to
promote healing from
within."

"My commitment to a
Hodgkin Lymphoma Diet
empowers me to take
control of my health."

CHAPTER 5: DINNER RECIPES

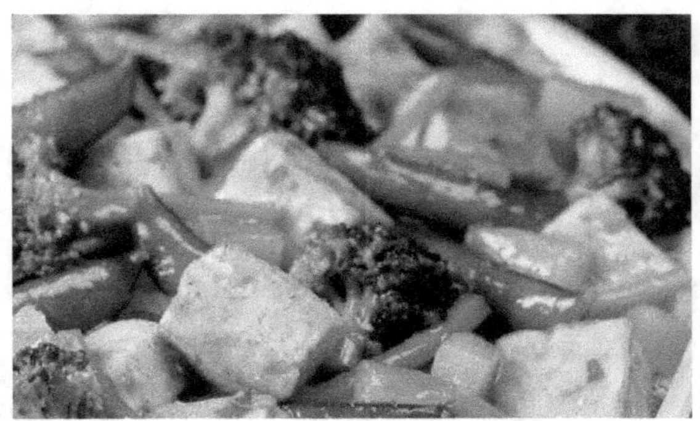

Salmon and Quinoa Stuffed Bell Peppers

Ingredients:

- 4 large bell peppers, halved and seeds removed
- 1 cup quinoa, rinsed and drained
- 2 cups water or vegetable broth
- 1 lb salmon filets, skinless and deboned
- 2 tablespoons olive oil, divided
- 1 small onion, finely chopped
- 2 cloves garlic, minced
- 1 teaspoon dried oregano
- 1 teaspoon dried thyme
- Salt and black pepper to taste
- 1 cup cherry tomatoes, halved

- 1/2 cup feta cheese, crumbled (optional)
- Fresh parsley for garnish

Instructions:

1. Preheat the oven to 375°F (190°C).

2. Place halved bell peppers in a baking dish and set aside.

3. In a medium saucepan, combine quinoa and water or vegetable broth. Bring to a boil, then reduce heat to low, cover, and simmer for 15-20 minutes or until the quinoa is cooked and water is absorbed. Fluff with a fork.

4. Season salmon fillets with salt and black pepper. Heat 1 tablespoon of olive oil in a skillet over medium heat. Cook the salmon for 3-4 minutes per side or until it flakes easily with a fork. Remove from heat and break into large flakes.

5. In the same skillet, add the remaining tablespoon of olive oil. Sauté chopped onion and minced garlic until softened.

6. Stir in dried oregano and dried thyme. Season with additional salt and black pepper if needed.

7. Combine the sautéed onion mixture with the cooked quinoa and flaked salmon in a bowl. Gently fold in the halved cherry tomatoes.

8. Stuff each bell pepper half with the salmon and quinoa mixture.

9. If using, sprinkle crumbled feta cheese over the stuffed peppers.

10. Bake in the preheated oven for 25-30 minutes or until the peppers are tender.

11. Garnish with fresh parsley before serving.

12. Serve your Salmon and Quinoa Stuffed Bell Peppers hot, and enjoy this flavorful and nutritious dish!

Vegetable and Lentil Curry

Ingredients:

- 1 cup dried green or brown lentils, rinsed and drained
- 2 tablespoons vegetable oil
- 1 large onion, finely chopped
- 3 cloves garlic, minced
- 1 tablespoon fresh ginger, grated
- 1 tablespoon curry powder
- 1 teaspoon ground cumin
- 1 teaspoon ground coriander
- 1/2 teaspoon turmeric
- 1/4 teaspoon cayenne pepper (adjust to taste)

- 1 can (14 oz) diced tomatoes
- 1 can (14 oz) coconut milk
- 4 cups mixed vegetables (e.g., carrots, bell peppers, zucchini, cauliflower), chopped
- Salt and black pepper to taste
- Fresh cilantro for garnish
- Cooked rice or naan for serving

Instructions:

1. In a medium saucepan, combine lentils with 3 cups of water. Bring to a boil, then reduce heat to low, cover, and simmer for 20-25 minutes or until the lentils are tender. Drain any excess water and set aside.

2. In a large pot or Dutch oven, heat vegetable oil over medium heat.

3. Add chopped onion, minced garlic, and grated ginger. Sauté for 3-4 minutes until the onions are soft and translucent.

4. Add curry powder, ground cumin, ground coriander, turmeric, and cayenne pepper (if using). Stir well to coat the onions in the spices and cook for an additional 2 minutes.

5. Pour in the diced tomatoes with their juice. Cook for 5 minutes, allowing the tomatoes to break down.

6. Stir in the cooked lentils and mixed vegetables. Mix well to coat the vegetables in the flavorful sauce.

7. Pour in the coconut milk and bring the curry to a simmer. Reduce the heat to low, cover, and let it cook for 15-20 minutes or until the vegetables are tender.

8. Season the vegetable and lentil curry with salt and black pepper to taste.

9. Taste and adjust the seasoning if necessary.

10. Serve the curry over cooked rice or with naan.

11. Garnish with fresh cilantro before serving.

12. Enjoy your wholesome and delicious Vegetable and Lentil Curry!

Grilled Turkey Burgers with Sweet Potato Wedges

Ingredients:

For the Turkey Burgers:

- 1 lb ground turkey
- 1/4 cup breadcrumbs

- 1/4 cup finely chopped onion

- 2 cloves garlic, minced

- 1 tablespoon Dijon mustard

- 1 tablespoon Worcestershire sauce

- 1 teaspoon dried thyme

- Salt and black pepper to taste

- Olive oil for grilling

For the Sweet Potato Wedges:

- 2 large sweet potatoes, peeled and cut into wedges

- 2 tablespoons olive oil

- 1 teaspoon paprika

- 1 teaspoon garlic powder

- 1 teaspoon dried rosemary

- Salt and black pepper to taste

For Serving:

- Whole wheat burger buns

- Lettuce leaves

- Sliced tomatoes

- Sliced red onion

- Mustard or your favorite burger condiments

Instructions:

For the Turkey Burgers:

1. In a large bowl, combine ground turkey, breadcrumbs, chopped onion, minced garlic, Dijon mustard, Worcestershire sauce, dried thyme, salt, and black pepper.
2. Mix the ingredients together until well combined, but avoid overmixing to keep the burgers tender.
3. Divide the mixture into four portions and shape them into burger patties.
4. Preheat the grill to medium-high heat.
5. Brush the turkey burgers with olive oil on both sides to prevent sticking.
6. Grill the turkey burgers for 5-6 minutes per side or until fully cooked and they reach an internal temperature of 165°F (74°C).
7. Toast the whole wheat burger buns on the grill for a minute or two until lightly browned.

For the Sweet Potato Wedges:

1. Preheat the oven to 400°F (200°C).
2. In a large bowl, toss sweet potato wedges with olive oil, paprika, garlic powder, dried rosemary, salt, and black pepper until evenly coated.

3. Spread the sweet potato wedges on a baking sheet lined with parchment paper.

4. Roast in the preheated oven for 25-30 minutes, flipping halfway through, until the sweet potatoes are tender and golden brown.

For Serving:

1. Assemble the grilled turkey burgers on the toasted buns with lettuce, sliced tomatoes, and red onion.

2. Serve alongside the roasted sweet potato wedges.

3. Add your favorite burger condiments like mustard or others of your choice.

4. Enjoy your Grilled Turkey Burgers with Sweet Potato Wedges!

Cauliflower and Chickpea Masala

Ingredients:

- 1 head cauliflower, cut into florets
- 1 can (14 oz) chickpeas, drained and rinsed
- 2 tablespoons vegetable oil
- 1 large onion, finely chopped
- 3 cloves garlic, minced
- 1 tablespoon fresh ginger, grated

- 1 tablespoon garam masala
- 1 teaspoon ground coriander
- 1 teaspoon ground cumin
- 1/2 teaspoon turmeric
- 1/4 teaspoon cayenne pepper (adjust to taste)
- 1 can (14 oz) diced tomatoes
- 1 can (14 oz) coconut milk
- Salt and black pepper to taste
- Fresh cilantro for garnish
- Cooked basmati rice or naan for serving

Instructions:

1. In a large pot or Dutch oven, heat vegetable oil over medium heat.

2. Add chopped onion, minced garlic, and grated ginger. Sauté for 3-4 minutes until the onions are soft and translucent.

3. Add garam masala, ground coriander, ground cumin, turmeric, and cayenne pepper (if using). Stir well to coat the onions in the spices and cook for an additional 2 minutes.

4. Add cauliflower florets and drained chickpeas to the pot. Stir to coat the vegetables in the flavorful spice mixture.

5. Pour in the diced tomatoes with their juice. Cook for 5 minutes, allowing the tomatoes to break down.

6. Stir in the coconut milk and bring the masala to a simmer. Reduce the heat to low, cover, and let it cook for 15-20 minutes or until the cauliflower is tender.

7. Season the cauliflower and chickpea masala with salt and black pepper to taste.

8. Taste and adjust the seasoning if necessary.

9. Serve the masala over cooked basmati rice or with naan.

10. Garnish with fresh cilantro before serving.

11. Enjoy your flavorful and aromatic Cauliflower and Chickpea Masala!

Baked Cod with Turmeric and Lemon

Ingredients:

- 4 cod filets (about 6 ounces each)
- 2 tablespoons olive oil
- 1 teaspoon ground turmeric
- 1 teaspoon paprika
- Salt and black pepper to taste
- Zest of 1 lemon

- Juice of 1 lemon
- 2 cloves garlic, minced
- Fresh parsley for garnish

Instructions:

1. Preheat your oven to 400°F (200°C).
2. Pat the cod filets dry with paper towels and place them in a baking dish.
3. In a small bowl, mix olive oil, ground turmeric, paprika, salt, black pepper, lemon zest, lemon juice, and minced garlic to create the marinade.
4. Pour the marinade over the cod filets, ensuring they are well coated. Allow the fish to marinate for at least 15-20 minutes.
5. Bake the cod in the preheated oven for 15-18 minutes or until the fish flakes easily with a fork and is opaque throughout.
6. While the cod is baking, you can baste it with the marinade halfway through cooking.
7. Once the cod is done, remove it from the oven and sprinkle with fresh parsley.
8. Serve the baked cod hot, perhaps with a side of steamed vegetables or a light salad.
9. Enjoy your light and flavorful Baked Cod with Turmeric and Lemon!

Miso-Glazed Tofu Stir-Fry

Ingredients:

For the Miso-Glazed Tofu:

- 1 block (14 oz) extra-firm tofu, pressed and cubed
- 3 tablespoons white miso paste
- 2 tablespoons soy sauce
- 1 tablespoon rice vinegar
- 1 tablespoon maple syrup or agave nectar
- 1 teaspoon sesame oil
- 2 cloves garlic, minced
- 1 teaspoon grated fresh ginger
- 2 tablespoons vegetable oil (for stir-frying)

For the Stir-Fry:

- 1 tablespoon vegetable oil
- 1 bell pepper, thinly sliced
- 1 carrot, julienned
- 1 cup broccoli florets
- 1 cup snow peas, ends trimmed
- 2 green onions, sliced
- Sesame seeds and sliced green onions for garnish
- Cooked brown rice or noodles for serving

Instructions:

For the Miso-Glazed Tofu:

1. In a bowl, whisk together miso paste, soy sauce, rice vinegar, maple syrup, sesame oil, minced garlic, and grated ginger to create the glaze.

2. Add the cubed tofu to the bowl and gently toss to coat the tofu in the miso glaze. Allow it to marinate for at least 15-20 minutes.

3. Heat 2 tablespoons of vegetable oil in a large skillet or wok over medium-high heat.

4. Add the marinated tofu to the skillet, spreading it out in a single layer. Cook for 3-4 minutes on each side or until golden brown and caramelized.

5. Remove the glazed tofu from the skillet and set aside.

For the Stir-Fry:

1. In the same skillet, add 1 tablespoon of vegetable oil over medium-high heat.

2. Add sliced bell pepper, julienned carrot, broccoli florets, and snow peas to the skillet. Stir-fry for 5-7 minutes or until the vegetables are tender-crisp.

3. Return the cooked miso-glazed tofu to the skillet, along with sliced green onions. Toss everything together to combine.

4. Cook for an additional 2-3 minutes until the tofu is heated through.

5. Serve the Miso-Glazed Tofu Stir-Fry over cooked brown rice or noodles.

6. Garnish with sesame seeds and additional sliced green onions.

7. Enjoy your delicious and flavorful Miso-Glazed Tofu Stir-Fry!

Chicken and Vegetable Skillet

Ingredients:

- 1 lb boneless, skinless chicken breasts, cut into bite-sized pieces
- 2 tablespoons olive oil
- 1 onion, thinly sliced
- 2 bell peppers, thinly sliced (any color)
- 2 zucchini, sliced
- 1 cup cherry tomatoes, halved
- 3 cloves garlic, minced
- 1 teaspoon dried thyme
- 1 teaspoon dried rosemary

- Salt and pepper to taste
- 1/2 cup chicken broth
- 2 tablespoons balsamic vinegar
- Fresh parsley for garnish

Instructions:

1. Heat 1 tablespoon of olive oil in a large skillet over medium-high heat.
2. Season the chicken pieces with salt and pepper, then add them to the skillet. Cook until browned on all sides and cooked through. Remove chicken from the skillet and set aside.
3. In the same skillet, add another tablespoon of olive oil. Add sliced onions and cook until they become translucent.
4. Add sliced bell peppers and zucchini to the skillet. Sauté until the vegetables are tender-crisp.
5. Stir in minced garlic, dried thyme, and dried rosemary. Sauté for an additional minute until the herbs become fragrant.
6. Return the cooked chicken to the skillet and add halved cherry tomatoes. Mix everything well.

7. Pour in chicken broth and balsamic vinegar. Stir to combine and let it simmer for a few minutes until the flavors meld.

8. Season with additional salt and pepper if needed. Adjust the balsamic vinegar to taste.

9. Once the vegetables are cooked to your liking, and the sauce has thickened slightly, remove the skillet from heat.

10. Garnish with fresh parsley before serving.

Spinach and Chickpea Salad with Grilled Chicken

Ingredients:

For the Salad:

- 1 lb boneless, skinless chicken breasts
- 1 can (15 oz) chickpeas, drained and rinsed
- 5 cups fresh baby spinach
- 1 cup cherry tomatoes, halved
- 1 cucumber, diced
- 1/2 red onion, thinly sliced
- 1/2 cup crumbled feta cheese (optional)
- 1/4 cup Kalamata olives, pitted and sliced (optional)

For the Grilled Chicken Marinade:

- 2 tablespoons olive oil
- 2 tablespoons lemon juice
- 2 cloves garlic, minced
- 1 teaspoon dried oregano
- Salt and pepper to taste

For the Dressing:

- 3 tablespoons olive oil
- 2 tablespoons balsamic vinegar
- 1 teaspoon Dijon mustard
- Salt and pepper to taste

Instructions:

1. In a bowl, combine the ingredients for the grilled chicken marinade. Add the chicken breasts, ensuring they are well-coated. Allow them to marinate for at least 30 minutes.

2. Preheat your grill or grill pan over medium-high heat. Grill the marinated chicken breasts for 6-8 minutes per side or until fully cooked. Let them rest for a few minutes before slicing.

3. In a large salad bowl, combine the baby spinach, cherry tomatoes, diced cucumber, sliced red onion, chickpeas, feta cheese, and Kalamata olives.

4. In a small bowl, whisk together the dressing ingredients - olive oil, balsamic vinegar, Dijon mustard, salt, and pepper.

5. Add the sliced grilled chicken to the salad.

6. Drizzle the dressing over the salad and toss everything gently to combine, ensuring the salad is evenly coated with the dressing.

7. Serve immediately, and enjoy your nutritious Spinach and Chickpea Salad with Grilled Chicken!

Quinoa and Black Bean Stuffed Peppers

Ingredients:

For the Stuffed Peppers:

- 4 large bell peppers, halved and seeds removed
- 1 cup quinoa, rinsed and cooked according to package instructions
- 1 can (15 oz) black beans, drained and rinsed
- 1 cup corn kernels (fresh or frozen)
- 1 cup diced tomatoes
- 1 cup shredded cheddar or Mexican blend cheese
- 1 teaspoon ground cumin

- 1 teaspoon chili powder
- 1/2 teaspoon garlic powder
- Salt and pepper to taste

For the Topping:

- 1 cup salsa
- 1/2 cup sour cream (optional)
- Fresh cilantro, chopped, for garnish

Instructions:

1. Preheat the oven to 375°F (190°C).
2. Place the halved bell peppers in a baking dish, cut side up.
3. In a large bowl, combine the cooked quinoa, black beans, corn, diced tomatoes, shredded cheese, ground cumin, chili powder, garlic powder, salt, and pepper. Mix well until all ingredients are evenly combined.
4. Stuff each bell pepper half with the quinoa and black bean mixture, pressing down gently to pack the filling.
5. Pour salsa over the stuffed peppers, covering them evenly.
6. Cover the baking dish with aluminum foil and bake in the preheated oven for 25-30 minutes, or until the peppers are tender.

7. Remove the foil and bake for an additional 5-10 minutes until the cheese on top is melted and bubbly.

8. Once done, remove from the oven and let them cool for a few minutes.

9. Serve the quinoa and black bean stuffed peppers topped with a dollop of sour cream (if using) and a sprinkle of fresh cilantro.

Roasted Vegetable and Lentil Bowl

Ingredients:

For the Roasted Vegetables:

- 1 large sweet potato, peeled and diced
- 2 carrots, peeled and sliced
- 1 zucchini, sliced
- 1 red bell pepper, sliced
- 1 red onion, thinly sliced
- 2 tablespoons olive oil
- 1 teaspoon dried thyme
- 1 teaspoon paprika
- Salt and pepper to taste

For the Lentils:

- 1 cup dry green or brown lentils, rinsed
- 3 cups vegetable broth or water

- 2 cloves garlic, minced

- 1 bay leaf

- Salt and pepper to taste

For the Tahini Dressing:

- 1/4 cup tahini

- 2 tablespoons lemon juice

- 1 tablespoon maple syrup or honey

- 1 clove garlic, minced

- 2 tablespoons water (or more for desired consistency)

- Salt and pepper to taste

For Assembly:

- Cooked quinoa or rice (optional)

Instructions:

1. Preheat the oven to 425°F (220°C).

2. Toss the sweet potato, carrots, zucchini, red bell pepper, and red onion in olive oil, dried thyme, paprika, salt, and pepper. Spread them out on a baking sheet in a single layer.

3. Roast the vegetables in the preheated oven for 25-30 minutes or until they are golden brown and tender, stirring once halfway through.

4. While the vegetables are roasting, prepare the lentils. In a medium saucepan, combine the lentils, vegetable broth or water, minced garlic, bay leaf, salt, and pepper. Bring to a boil, then reduce the heat to low, cover, and simmer for about 20-25 minutes or until the lentils are tender. Drain any excess liquid.

5. In a small bowl, whisk together the tahini, lemon juice, maple syrup or honey, minced garlic, water, salt, and pepper to create the dressing.

6. Once the vegetables and lentils are ready, assemble your bowls. Start with a base of cooked quinoa or rice if using.

7. Top the grains with a generous portion of roasted vegetables and lentils.

8. Drizzle the tahini dressing over the bowl.

9. Garnish with fresh herbs or additional seasoning if desired.

Turkey and Quinoa Casserole

Ingredients:

- 1 lb ground turkey
- 1 cup quinoa, rinsed
- 1 onion, finely chopped

- 2 cloves garlic, minced
- 1 bell pepper, diced
- 1 zucchini, diced
- 1 cup frozen peas
- 1 can (14 oz) diced tomatoes, drained
- 1 teaspoon dried thyme
- 1 teaspoon dried oregano
- 1 teaspoon ground cumin
- Salt and pepper to taste
- 2 cups chicken or vegetable broth
- 1 cup shredded cheddar cheese
- Fresh parsley, chopped, for garnish (optional)

Instructions:

1. Preheat the oven to 375°F (190°C).
2. In a large skillet, cook the ground turkey over medium heat until browned. Drain any excess fat.
3. Add chopped onion and minced garlic to the skillet, sautéing until the onion is translucent.
4. Stir in diced bell pepper and zucchini, cooking for an additional 3-5 minutes until the vegetables begin to soften.

5. Add quinoa, frozen peas, diced tomatoes, dried thyme, dried oregano, ground cumin, salt, and pepper to the skillet. Mix well to combine.

6. Pour in the chicken or vegetable broth and bring the mixture to a simmer. Allow it to simmer for about 10 minutes, ensuring the quinoa is partially cooked.

7. Transfer the mixture to a greased casserole dish.

8. Sprinkle shredded cheddar cheese over the top of the casserole.

9. Cover the casserole dish with aluminum foil and bake in the preheated oven for 25-30 minutes or until the quinoa is fully cooked and the cheese is melted and bubbly.

10. Remove the foil during the last 10 minutes of baking to allow the cheese to brown slightly.

11. Once done, remove from the oven and let it rest for a few minutes before serving.

12. Garnish with chopped fresh parsley if desired.

Sweet Potato and Kale Hash with Poached Eggs

Ingredients:

- 2 large sweet potatoes, peeled and diced

- 1 bunch kale, stems removed and leaves chopped
- 1 onion, finely chopped
- 2 cloves garlic, minced
- 2 tablespoons olive oil
- 1 teaspoon smoked paprika
- 1/2 teaspoon cumin
- Salt and pepper to taste
- 4 large eggs
- Chopped fresh parsley for garnish (optional)

Instructions:

1. In a large skillet, heat olive oil over medium heat.

2. Add the chopped onion and sauté until it becomes translucent.

3. Add the diced sweet potatoes to the skillet. Cook for about 10-15 minutes, stirring occasionally, until the sweet potatoes are tender and slightly browned.

4. Add minced garlic, smoked paprika, cumin, salt, and pepper to the skillet. Stir to coat the sweet potatoes evenly with the spices.

5. Add the chopped kale to the skillet. Cook for an additional 5-7 minutes until the kale is wilted and tender.

6. Create four wells in the sweet potato and kale mixture for the poached eggs.

7. Crack one egg into each well. Cover the skillet and let the eggs poach for about 5-7 minutes or until the egg whites are set but the yolks are still runny.

8. Once the eggs are poached to your liking, remove the skillet from heat.

9. Garnish with chopped fresh parsley if desired.

10. Serve the Sweet Potato and Kale Hash with Poached Eggs immediately, and enjoy this nutritious and delicious breakfast or brunch dish!

CHAPTER 6: SNACKS AND APPETIZERS

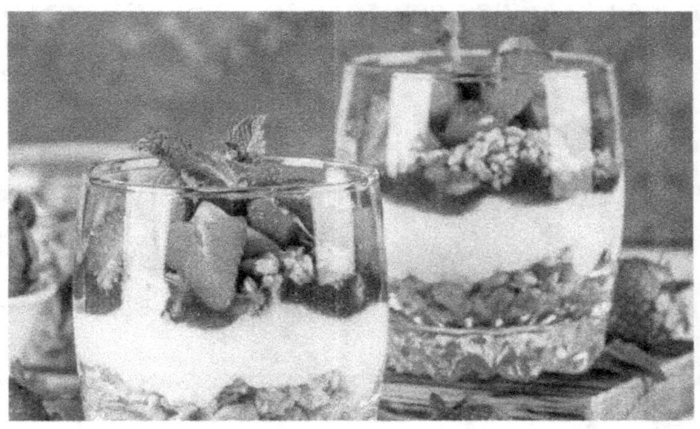

SNACKS

Greek Yogurt Parfait with Berries

Ingredients:

- 1 cup Greek yogurt (unsweetened)
- 1 cup mixed berries (strawberries, blueberries, raspberries)
- 1/4 cup granola
- 1 tablespoon honey or maple syrup (optional)
- 1/2 teaspoon vanilla extract
- Fresh mint leaves for garnish (optional)

Instructions:

1. In a bowl, mix Greek yogurt with vanilla extract. If you prefer a sweeter taste, add honey or maple syrup to the yogurt and stir until well combined.
2. Wash and prepare the berries. If using strawberries, hull and slice them.
3. Begin layering your parfait. In serving glasses or bowls, start with a spoonful of Greek yogurt at the bottom.
4. Add a layer of mixed berries on top of the yogurt.
5. Sprinkle a layer of granola over the berries. This adds a crunchy texture to the parfait.
6. Repeat the layers until you fill the serving glasses or bowls, finishing with a dollop of Greek yogurt on top.
7. Drizzle honey or maple syrup over the final layer if you want a touch of sweetness.
8. Garnish with fresh mint leaves for a burst of freshness and added aroma.
9. Serve immediately and enjoy your delicious and nutritious Greek Yogurt Parfait with Berries!

Turmeric Hummus with Veggie Sticks

Ingredients:

For Turmeric Hummus:

- 1 can (15 oz) chickpeas, drained and rinsed
- 1/4 cup tahini
- 2 tablespoons olive oil
- 2 cloves garlic, minced
- 1 teaspoon ground turmeric
- 1 teaspoon ground cumin
- 1/2 teaspoon ground coriander
- Juice of 1 lemon
- Salt and pepper to taste
- 2-3 tablespoons water (for desired consistency)

For Veggie Sticks:

- Carrot sticks
- Cucumber sticks
- Bell pepper strips (any color)
- Cherry tomatoes, halved
- Celery sticks

Instructions:

For Turmeric Hummus:

1. In a food processor, combine chickpeas, tahini, olive oil, minced garlic, ground turmeric, ground cumin, ground coriander, lemon juice, salt, and pepper.

2. Blend the ingredients until smooth, scraping down the sides of the processor as needed.

3. If the hummus is too thick, add water a tablespoon at a time until you reach your desired consistency.

4. Adjust salt, pepper, and lemon juice to taste.

5. Transfer the turmeric hummus to a serving bowl.

For Veggie Sticks:

1. Wash and prepare the vegetables for dipping. Cut carrots, cucumber, bell peppers, cherry tomatoes, and celery into sticks or strips.

2. Arrange the veggie sticks around the turmeric hummus bowl for a colorful presentation.

3. Serve immediately and enjoy your Turmeric Hummus with Veggie Sticks as a healthy and flavorful snack!

Almond Butter and Banana Bites

Ingredients:

- 2 large bananas, peeled and sliced into rounds
- Almond butter (or any nut butter of your choice)
- Chia seeds (optional)
- Unsweetened shredded coconut (optional)
- Sliced almonds (optional)

- Honey or maple syrup for drizzling (optional)

Instructions:

1. Lay the banana slices on a flat surface or a serving plate.

2. Spread a small amount of almond butter on top of each banana round. You can use the back of a spoon for easy spreading.

3. Optionally, sprinkle chia seeds, shredded coconut, and sliced almonds on top of the almond butter.

4. Drizzle a bit of honey or maple syrup over the banana rounds for added sweetness, if desired.

5. If serving immediately, enjoy your Almond Butter and Banana Bites as a tasty snack or light dessert.

6. If not serving immediately, refrigerate the bites for a short period to prevent browning of the bananas.

Roasted Chickpeas with Herbs

Ingredients:

- 2 cans (15 oz each) chickpeas, drained and rinsed
- 2 tablespoons olive oil

- 1 teaspoon garlic powder
- 1 teaspoon onion powder
- 1 teaspoon dried oregano
- 1 teaspoon dried thyme
- 1/2 teaspoon smoked paprika
- 1/2 teaspoon cayenne pepper (adjust to taste)
- Salt and pepper to taste

Instructions:

1. Preheat the oven to 400°F (200°C) and line a baking sheet with parchment paper.

2. Rinse and drain the chickpeas, then pat them dry with a paper towel to remove excess moisture.

3. In a bowl, toss the chickpeas with olive oil, garlic powder, onion powder, dried oregano, dried thyme, smoked paprika, cayenne pepper, salt, and pepper. Ensure the chickpeas are evenly coated.

4. Spread the seasoned chickpeas in a single layer on the prepared baking sheet.

5. Roast in the preheated oven for 25-30 minutes, shaking the pan or stirring the chickpeas halfway through the cooking time. The chickpeas should be golden brown and crispy.

6. Remove from the oven and let them cool slightly before serving.

7. Taste and adjust the seasoning if necessary. Add more salt, pepper, or herbs according to your preference.

8. Serve the Roasted Chickpeas with Herbs as a crunchy and flavorful snack or use them as a topping for salads or soups.

Avocado and Tomato Salsa on Whole Grain Crackers

Ingredients:

- 2 ripe avocados, diced
- 1 cup cherry tomatoes, diced
- 1/4 cup red onion, finely chopped
- 1/4 cup fresh cilantro, chopped
- 1 jalapeño, seeded and finely chopped (optional for heat)
- Juice of 1 lime
- Salt and pepper to taste
- Whole grain crackers for serving

Instructions:

1. In a medium-sized bowl, combine diced avocados, cherry tomatoes, red onion, cilantro, and jalapeño (if using).
2. Squeeze the juice of one lime over the mixture to add a burst of citrus flavor.
3. Gently toss the ingredients together until well combined.
4. Season the avocado and tomato salsa with salt and pepper to taste. Adjust the seasoning according to your preference.
5. Allow the salsa to sit for a few minutes to let the flavors meld.
6. Just before serving, give the salsa a final gentle toss.
7. Spoon the Avocado and Tomato Salsa onto whole grain crackers, distributing it evenly.
8. Serve immediately and enjoy this refreshing and flavorful snack!

Mixed Nuts and Dried Fruits

Ingredients:

- 1 cup almonds
- 1 cup walnuts

- 1 cup cashews
- 1 cup pistachios
- 1 cup mixed dried fruits (apricots, cranberries, raisins, etc.)
- 2 tablespoons melted butter
- 2 tablespoons honey
- 1 teaspoon cinnamon
- 1/2 teaspoon sea salt

Instructions:

1. Preheat the oven to 350°F (175°C) and line a baking sheet with parchment paper.
2. In a large bowl, combine the almonds, walnuts, cashews, and pistachios.
3. In a small bowl, mix together the melted butter, honey, cinnamon, and sea salt until well combined.
4. Pour the honey mixture over the mixed nuts and toss until all the nuts are evenly coated.
5. Spread the coated nuts in a single layer on the prepared baking sheet.
6. Bake in the preheated oven for about 15-20 minutes, or until the nuts are golden brown and fragrant. Stir the nuts halfway through the baking time for even toasting.

7. Remove the baking sheet from the oven and let the nuts cool completely.

8. Once the nuts are cooled, add the mixed dried fruits and toss to combine.

9. Store the mixed nuts and dried fruits in an airtight container. Enjoy as a snack or add them to your favorite dishes.

Cucumber and Hummus Roll-Ups

Ingredients:

- 1 large cucumber
- 1 cup hummus (store-bought or homemade)
- 1/2 cup cherry tomatoes, diced
- 1/4 cup red onion, finely chopped
- 1/4 cup feta cheese, crumbled (optional)
- 1 tablespoon fresh dill, chopped
- Salt and pepper to taste

Instructions:

1. Wash the cucumber thoroughly and trim off the ends. Using a vegetable peeler, slice the cucumber lengthwise into thin strips or use a mandolin for even slices.

2. Lay the cucumber slices on a clean surface or cutting board. Pat them dry with a paper towel to remove excess moisture.

3. Spread a thin layer of hummus onto each cucumber slice, leaving a small border around the edges.

4. Sprinkle diced cherry tomatoes, chopped red onion, crumbled feta cheese (if using), and fresh dill evenly over the hummus layer.

5. Season with salt and pepper to taste.

6. Carefully roll up each cucumber slice, starting from one end and securing it with a toothpick if needed.

7. Arrange the cucumber and hummus roll-ups on a serving platter.

8. Optional: Chill in the refrigerator for about 30 minutes before serving to enhance the flavors and firm up the rolls.

9. Serve the cucumber and hummus roll-ups as a refreshing appetizer or a healthy snack.

Chia Seed Pudding with Mango

Ingredients:

- 1/4 cup chia seeds

- 1 cup almond milk (or any milk of your choice)
- 1 tablespoon maple syrup or honey
- 1/2 teaspoon vanilla extract
- 1 ripe mango, peeled and diced
- Optional toppings: sliced almonds, shredded coconut, or mint leaves

Instructions:

1. In a mixing bowl, combine chia seeds, almond milk, maple syrup (or honey), and vanilla extract. Stir well to ensure the chia seeds are evenly distributed.

2. Let the mixture sit for about 5 minutes, and then stir again to prevent clumping. Repeat this process a couple of times within the first 15-20 minutes.

3. Cover the bowl and refrigerate the chia seed mixture for at least 3 hours or preferably overnight. This allows the chia seeds to absorb the liquid and create a pudding-like consistency.

4. Before serving, give the chia pudding a good stir to break up any clumps that may have formed. If it's too thick, you can add a little more almond milk to reach your desired consistency.

5. In a separate bowl, dice the ripe mango into small, bite-sized pieces.

6. Layer the chia seed pudding and diced mango in serving glasses or bowls.

7. Optional: Top the pudding with sliced almonds, shredded coconut, or garnish with mint leaves for added flavor and texture.

8. Serve chilled and enjoy this healthy and delicious chia seed pudding with mango!

Edamame with Sea Salt

Ingredients:

- 2 cups fresh or frozen edamame in pods
- 1 tablespoon sea salt
- Water for boiling

Instructions:

1. If using frozen edamame, thaw them according to the package instructions.

2. In a large pot, bring water to a boil. Add a generous pinch of salt to the boiling water.

3. Add the edamame pods to the boiling water. Cook for about 3-5 minutes, or until the edamame pods are tender.

4. Drain the edamame in a colander and transfer them to a large bowl.

5. While the edamame are still hot, sprinkle them with sea salt. Toss the edamame gently to ensure the salt is evenly distributed.

6. Allow the edamame to cool for a few minutes before serving. They can be served warm or at room temperature.

7. To eat, simply squeeze the edamame pod at one end, and the beans will pop out into your mouth. Discard the empty pods.

8. Optionally, you can serve the edamame with an additional side of sea salt for dipping.

Whole Grain Toast with Ricotta and Berries

Ingredients:

- 4 slices of whole grain bread
- 1 cup ricotta cheese
- 1 cup mixed berries (strawberries, blueberries, raspberries)
- 2 tablespoons honey
- Fresh mint leaves for garnish (optional)

Instructions:

1. Toast the whole grain bread slices to your desired level of crispiness.

2. While the bread is toasting, wash and prepare the berries. If using strawberries, hull and slice them.

3. Once the toast is ready, let it cool for a minute or two.

4. Spread a generous layer of ricotta cheese onto each slice of toasted bread.

5. Arrange the mixed berries on top of the ricotta, distributing them evenly among the slices.

6. Drizzle honey over the berries and ricotta. Adjust the amount of honey to your sweetness preference.

7. Optionally, garnish with fresh mint leaves for added freshness.

8. Serve the whole grain toast with ricotta and berries immediately, while the toast is still warm.

Sliced Apple with Almond Butter

Ingredients:

- 2 medium-sized apples (any variety you prefer)

- 1/4 cup almond butter
- 1 tablespoon honey (optional)
- 1 tablespoon chia seeds (optional)
- A sprinkle of cinnamon (optional)

Instructions:

1. Wash the apples thoroughly and slice them into thin rounds or wedges, removing the core and seeds.

2. Arrange the apple slices on a serving plate or platter.

3. In a small microwave-safe bowl, warm the almond butter for a few seconds until it becomes slightly more fluid, making it easier to drizzle.

4. Drizzle the almond butter over the apple slices. You can use a spoon or a small plastic bag with the tip snipped off for a more controlled drizzle.

5. Optional: Drizzle honey over the apple slices for added sweetness.

6. Optionally, sprinkle chia seeds over the almond butter for a nutritional boost and added texture.

7. If desired, finish with a light sprinkle of cinnamon for extra flavor.

8. Serve immediately and enjoy this simple, nutritious, and satisfying snack or breakfast option.

Kale Chips with Lemon and Parmesan

Ingredients:

- 1 bunch of fresh kale
- 1 tablespoon olive oil
- 1 tablespoon fresh lemon juice
- 1/4 cup grated Parmesan cheese
- Salt and pepper to taste

Instructions:

1. Preheat your oven to 350°F (175°C).
2. Wash the kale thoroughly and pat it dry with a clean kitchen towel. Remove the tough stems and tear the kale leaves into bite-sized pieces.
3. In a large bowl, toss the kale with olive oil, ensuring that the leaves are evenly coated.
4. Spread the kale pieces in a single layer on a baking sheet lined with parchment paper.
5. Bake in the preheated oven for about 10-15 minutes or until the edges of the kale are crispy but not burnt. Keep a close eye on them, as cooking times may vary based on your oven.

6. While the kale chips are still warm, drizzle them with fresh lemon juice.

7. Sprinkle grated Parmesan cheese over the kale chips, distributing it evenly.

8. Season with salt and pepper to taste. Toss the kale gently to combine all the flavors.

9. Allow the kale chips to cool for a few minutes before serving.

10. Serve the lemon and Parmesan kale chips as a healthy snack or a crunchy side dish.

APPETIZERS

Turmeric and Ginger Spiced Edamame

Ingredients:

- 2 cups fresh or frozen edamame in pods
- 1 tablespoon olive oil
- 1 teaspoon ground turmeric
- 1 teaspoon ground ginger
- 1/2 teaspoon garlic powder
- 1/2 teaspoon cumin
- 1/2 teaspoon smoked paprika
- Salt to taste
- Fresh cilantro for garnish (optional)

Instructions:

1. If using frozen edamame, thaw them according to the package instructions.

2. In a large pot, bring water to a boil. Add a generous pinch of salt to the boiling water.

3. Add the edamame pods to the boiling water. Cook for about 3-5 minutes, or until the edamame pods are tender.

4. While the edamame is cooking, prepare the spice mixture. In a small bowl, combine ground turmeric, ground ginger, garlic powder, cumin, smoked paprika, and a pinch of salt. Mix well.

5. Drain the edamame in a colander and transfer them to a large bowl.

6. In a large skillet, heat olive oil over medium heat.

7. Add the spice mixture to the skillet and sauté for about 30 seconds, stirring constantly to prevent burning.

8. Add the cooked edamame to the skillet, tossing them to coat evenly with the spice mixture. Sauté for an additional 2-3 minutes.

9. Optional: Garnish the spiced edamame with fresh cilantro for added freshness.

10. Serve the turmeric and ginger spiced edamame warm as a flavorful and nutritious snack or appetizer.

Mango Avocado Salsa

Ingredients:

- 1 ripe mango, peeled, pitted, and diced
- 1 ripe avocado, peeled, pitted, and diced
- 1/2 cup red onion, finely chopped
- 1/2 cup cherry tomatoes, diced
- 1/4 cup fresh cilantro, chopped
- 1 jalapeño, seeds removed and finely chopped (adjust to taste)
- 1 lime, juiced
- Salt and pepper to taste

Instructions:

1. In a large bowl, combine diced mango, diced avocado, chopped red onion, diced cherry tomatoes, and chopped cilantro.
2. Add finely chopped jalapeño to the bowl. Adjust the amount according to your desired level of spiciness.

3. Squeeze the juice of one lime over the mixture. The lime juice not only adds flavor but also helps prevent the avocado from browning.

4. Gently toss all the ingredients together until well combined.

5. Season the mango avocado salsa with salt and pepper to taste. Mix again to distribute the seasoning evenly.

6. Taste the salsa and adjust the lime, salt, or pepper if needed.

7. Cover the bowl with plastic wrap and refrigerate for at least 30 minutes to allow the flavors to meld.

8. Before serving, give the salsa a final gentle stir.

9. Serve the mango avocado salsa as a refreshing topping for grilled chicken, fish, tacos, or as a dip with tortilla chips.

Quinoa Stuffed Mini Bell Peppers

Ingredients:

- 1 cup quinoa, rinsed and cooked according to package instructions
- 12-15 mini bell peppers, halved and seeds removed

- 1 cup black beans, drained and rinsed
- 1 cup corn kernels (fresh, frozen, or canned)
- 1 cup cherry tomatoes, diced
- 1/2 cup red onion, finely chopped
- 1/4 cup fresh cilantro, chopped
- 1 teaspoon ground cumin
- 1 teaspoon chili powder
- 1/2 teaspoon garlic powder
- Salt and pepper to taste
- 1 cup shredded cheese (cheddar or Mexican blend)
- Optional toppings: sliced green onions, avocado, sour cream

Instructions:

1. Preheat the oven to 375°F (190°C).
2. Cook quinoa according to package instructions and set aside.
3. Cut the mini bell peppers in half lengthwise, remove seeds, and place them on a baking sheet.
4. In a large mixing bowl, combine cooked quinoa, black beans, corn, diced cherry tomatoes, red onion, chopped cilantro, ground cumin, chili powder, garlic powder, salt, and pepper. Mix well to combine.

5. Spoon the quinoa mixture into each halved mini bell pepper, pressing it down slightly.

6. Sprinkle shredded cheese over the stuffed peppers, covering the filling.

7. Bake in the preheated oven for 15-20 minutes or until the peppers are tender, and the cheese is melted and bubbly.

8. Optional: Broil for an additional 1-2 minutes to achieve a golden brown top.

9. Remove from the oven and let them cool for a few minutes.

10. Garnish with optional toppings like sliced green onions, avocado, and a dollop of sour cream.

11. Serve the quinoa-stuffed mini bell peppers as a flavorful and nutritious appetizer or side dish.

Cucumber Dill Greek Yogurt Dip

Ingredients:

- 1 cup Greek yogurt
- 1/2 cucumber, finely diced
- 1 tablespoon fresh dill, chopped
- 1 clove garlic, minced
- 1 tablespoon lemon juice
- Salt and pepper to taste

Instructions:

1. Start by finely dicing the cucumber. If the cucumber has a lot of moisture, you may want to pat it dry with a paper towel to prevent the dip from becoming too watery.

2. In a medium-sized mixing bowl, combine Greek yogurt, diced cucumber, chopped fresh dill, minced garlic, and lemon juice.

3. Stir the ingredients together until well combined.

4. Season the cucumber dill Greek yogurt dip with salt and pepper to taste. Mix again and adjust the seasoning if needed.

5. Cover the bowl with plastic wrap and refrigerate the dip for at least 30 minutes to allow the flavors to meld.

6. Before serving, give the dip a final stir.

7. Optional: Garnish with additional fresh dill before serving.

8. Serve the cucumber dill Greek yogurt dip with vegetable sticks, pita bread, or as a refreshing condiment for grilled meats.

Smoked Salmon Cucumber Bites

Ingredients:

- 1 English cucumber, sliced into rounds
- 4 ounces smoked salmon, thinly sliced
- 1/2 cup cream cheese, softened
- 1 tablespoon fresh dill, chopped
- 1 tablespoon capers, drained
- 1 teaspoon lemon zest
- Freshly ground black pepper, to taste
- Chives or green onions for garnish (optional)

Instructions:

1. In a small bowl, mix together the softened cream cheese and chopped fresh dill until well combined.
2. Lay out the cucumber slices on a serving platter or tray.
3. Spread a thin layer of the cream cheese and dill mixture onto each cucumber round.
4. Place a small piece of smoked salmon on top of the cream cheese layer, ensuring it covers the cucumber.
5. Sprinkle capers evenly over the smoked salmon layer.

6. Zest a lemon, and then sprinkle the lemon zest over the top of the smoked salmon.

7. Finish with a touch of freshly ground black pepper for added flavor.

8. Optional: Garnish each smoked salmon cucumber bite with chives or thinly sliced green onions.

9. Arrange the smoked salmon cucumber bites on a serving platter and refrigerate until ready to serve.

10. Serve chilled as an elegant appetizer for parties or gatherings.

Roasted Garlic Hummus with Crudites

Ingredients:

For Roasted Garlic Hummus:

- 1 can (15 ounces) chickpeas, drained and rinsed
- 1/4 cup tahini
- 1/4 cup extra-virgin olive oil
- 1 head of garlic
- 1 lemon, juiced
- 1/2 teaspoon ground cumin
- Salt and pepper to taste
- Water (as needed for consistency)

For Crudites:

- An assortment of fresh vegetables such as carrots, cucumber, bell peppers, and cherry tomatoes, washed and cut into bite-sized pieces

Instructions:

For Roasted Garlic Hummus:

1. Preheat the oven to 400°F (200°C).

2. Cut off the top of the garlic head to expose the cloves. Place the garlic head on a piece of foil, drizzle with olive oil, and wrap it in the foil.

3. Roast the garlic in the preheated oven for about 30-40 minutes or until the cloves are soft and golden. Allow it to cool.

4. In a food processor, combine the drained chickpeas, tahini, extra-virgin olive oil, lemon juice, cumin, and roasted garlic cloves (squeeze the soft cloves out of the skin).

5. Process the mixture until smooth, scraping down the sides of the food processor as needed.

6. Season the hummus with salt and pepper to taste. If the consistency is too thick, you can add water, one tablespoon at a time, until you reach your desired texture.

7. Transfer the roasted garlic hummus to a serving bowl.

For Crudites:

8. Prepare an assortment of fresh vegetables such as carrots, cucumber, bell peppers, and cherry tomatoes. Cut them into bite-sized pieces or strips.

9. Arrange the crudites around the bowl of roasted garlic hummus on a serving platter.

10. Optionally, drizzle a little extra-virgin olive oil on top of the hummus and garnish with a sprinkle of cumin or chopped fresh herbs.

11. Serve the roasted garlic hummus with crudites as a tasty and healthy appetizer or snack.

Caprese Skewers with Balsamic Glaze

Ingredients:

- Cherry tomatoes
- Fresh mozzarella balls (bocconcini)
- Fresh basil leaves
- Balsamic glaze
- Wooden skewers

Instructions:

1. Begin by soaking the wooden skewers in water for about 30 minutes. This helps prevent them from splintering or burning during cooking.
2. Assemble the ingredients: cherry tomatoes, fresh mozzarella balls, and fresh basil leaves.
3. To make a Caprese skewer, thread one cherry tomato onto the skewer, followed by a folded basil leaf, and then a mozzarella ball. Repeat this pattern until the skewer is filled, leaving a small space at the end for easy handling.
4. Repeat the process until you have the desired number of Caprese skewers.
5. Arrange the skewers on a serving platter or plate.
6. Drizzle balsamic glaze over the Caprese skewers. You can either use store-bought balsamic glaze or make your own by reducing balsamic vinegar on the stove until it thickens.
7. Optionally, sprinkle a pinch of salt and pepper over the skewers for added flavor.
8. Serve the Caprese skewers immediately as a delightful appetizer or party snack.

Spicy Kale Chips

Ingredients:

- 1 bunch of kale
- 2 tablespoons olive oil
- 1 teaspoon chili powder
- 1/2 teaspoon smoked paprika
- 1/4 teaspoon cayenne pepper (adjust to taste)
- 1/2 teaspoon garlic powder
- Salt to taste

Instructions:

1. Preheat your oven to 300°F (150°C). Line a baking sheet with parchment paper.
2. Wash the kale thoroughly and pat it dry with a clean kitchen towel. Remove the tough stems and tear the kale leaves into bite-sized pieces.
3. In a large bowl, combine the kale pieces with olive oil. Toss to ensure that the kale leaves are evenly coated.
4. In a small bowl, mix together chili powder, smoked paprika, cayenne pepper, garlic powder, and salt.
5. Sprinkle the spice mixture over the kale, tossing the leaves to evenly distribute the spices.

6. Spread the kale pieces in a single layer on the prepared baking sheet. Avoid overcrowding to ensure crispy results.

7. Bake in the preheated oven for approximately 20-25 minutes or until the kale chips are crispy and the edges are slightly browned. Keep a close eye on them, as cooking times may vary.

8. Allow the spicy kale chips to cool on the baking sheet for a few minutes before transferring them to a serving bowl or plate.

9. Serve the chips as a spicy and nutritious snack or a crunchy side.

Turmeric Deviled Eggs

Ingredients:
- 6 large eggs
- 3 tablespoons mayonnaise
- 1 teaspoon Dijon mustard
- 1 teaspoon white vinegar
- 1/2 teaspoon ground turmeric
- 1/4 teaspoon smoked paprika
- Salt and pepper to taste
- Fresh cilantro or chives for garnish (optional)

Instructions:

1. Place the eggs in a single layer in a saucepan and cover them with water. Bring the water to a boil, then reduce the heat to low and simmer for 10-12 minutes.

2. Drain the eggs and transfer them to a bowl of ice water to cool. Once cooled, peel the eggs and cut them in half lengthwise.

3. Gently scoop out the yolks and place them in a separate bowl. Set the egg white halves aside.

4. Mash the egg yolks with a fork, and then add mayonnaise, Dijon mustard, white vinegar, ground turmeric, smoked paprika, salt, and pepper. Mix until smooth and well combined.

5. Adjust the seasoning to taste, adding more salt, pepper, or other spices if desired.

6. Spoon or pipe the yolk mixture back into the egg white halves.

7. Optional: Garnish each turmeric deviled egg with fresh cilantro or chives for a burst of color and added flavor.

8. Refrigerate the deviled eggs for at least 30 minutes to allow the flavors to meld.

9. Serve chilled as a colorful and flavorful appetizer.

Beet and Walnut Spread with Whole Grain Crackers

Ingredients:

For Beet and Walnut Spread:

- 2 medium-sized beets, roasted and peeled
- 1/2 cup walnuts, toasted
- 2 tablespoons olive oil
- 1 tablespoon balsamic vinegar
- 1 clove garlic, minced
- Salt and pepper to taste

For Whole Grain Crackers:

- Whole grain crackers of your choice

Instructions:

For Beet and Walnut Spread:

1. Preheat the oven to 400°F (200°C).
2. Wash the beets, trim the ends, and wrap them individually in foil. Place them on a baking sheet.
3. Roast the beets in the preheated oven for about 45-60 minutes or until they are tender when pierced with a fork.

4. Once roasted, let the beets cool slightly before peeling. The skins should easily slide off.

5. In a food processor, combine the roasted and peeled beets, toasted walnuts, olive oil, balsamic vinegar, minced garlic, salt, and pepper.

6. Process the mixture until smooth, scraping down the sides of the food processor as needed.

7. Taste the beet and walnut spread and adjust the seasoning if necessary.

8. Transfer the spread to a serving bowl.

For Whole Grain Crackers:

9. Arrange the whole grain crackers on a serving platter.

10. Serve the beet and walnut spread alongside the whole grain crackers.

11. Optionally, garnish the spread with additional toasted walnuts or a drizzle of balsamic vinegar for added flair.

Tomato Basil Bruschetta

Ingredients:

- 4-5 ripe tomatoes, diced
- 1/2 cup fresh basil leaves, chopped
- 3 cloves garlic, minced

- 2 tablespoons extra-virgin olive oil
- 1 tablespoon balsamic vinegar
- Salt and pepper to taste
- Baguette or Italian bread, sliced

Instructions:

1. In a large bowl, combine the diced tomatoes, chopped fresh basil, minced garlic, extra-virgin olive oil, and balsamic vinegar.

2. Gently toss the ingredients together until well mixed.

3. Season the tomato basil mixture with salt and pepper to taste. Mix again and adjust the seasoning if necessary.

4. Allow the bruschetta mixture to sit for at least 15-20 minutes at room temperature. This helps the flavors meld together.

5. While the mixture is resting, preheat your oven broiler or grill.

6. Arrange the sliced baguette or Italian bread on a baking sheet.

7. Toast the bread under the broiler or on the grill for 1-2 minutes per side or until golden and slightly crispy.

8. Once the bread is toasted, remove it from the oven or grill.

9. Just before serving, spoon the tomato basil mixture generously onto each slice of toasted bread.

10. Optionally, drizzle a little extra olive oil over the top and garnish with additional fresh basil leaves.

11. Serve the tomato basil bruschetta immediately as a delicious appetizer.

Avocado Cilantro Lime Shrimp Cocktail

Ingredients:

For Shrimp:

- 1 pound large shrimp, peeled and deveined
- 1 tablespoon olive oil
- Salt and pepper to taste

For Avocado Cilantro Lime Sauce:

- 2 ripe avocados, peeled and pitted
- 1/4 cup fresh cilantro, chopped
- 1/4 cup red onion, finely chopped
- 2 cloves garlic, minced
- Juice of 2 limes

- 1 tablespoon olive oil

- Salt and pepper to taste

For Shrimp Cocktail:

- Cocktail sauce (store-bought or homemade)

- Lime wedges for garnish

- Fresh cilantro leaves for garnish

Instructions:

For Shrimp:

1. In a large skillet, heat olive oil over medium-high heat.

2. Season the peeled and deveined shrimp with salt and pepper.

3. Cook the shrimp in the heated skillet for 2-3 minutes per side or until they are opaque and cooked through. Set aside.

For Avocado Cilantro Lime Sauce:

4. In a food processor or blender, combine the peeled and pitted avocados, chopped cilantro, finely chopped red onion, minced garlic, lime juice, and olive oil.

5. Process the ingredients until smooth, scraping down the sides of the processor or blender as needed.

6. Season the avocado cilantro lime sauce with salt and pepper to taste. Adjust the seasoning if necessary.

For Shrimp Cocktail:

7. In serving glasses or bowls, spoon a layer of cocktail sauce.

8. Place a few cooked shrimp on top of the cocktail sauce.

9. Spoon the avocado cilantro lime sauce generously over the shrimp and cocktail sauce.

10. Garnish the shrimp cocktail with lime wedges and fresh cilantro leaves.

11. Optionally, serve with additional lime wedges on the side.

12. Serve the avocado cilantro lime shrimp cocktail immediately as a refreshing and flavorful appetizer.

CHAPTER 7: HERBS AND SPICES

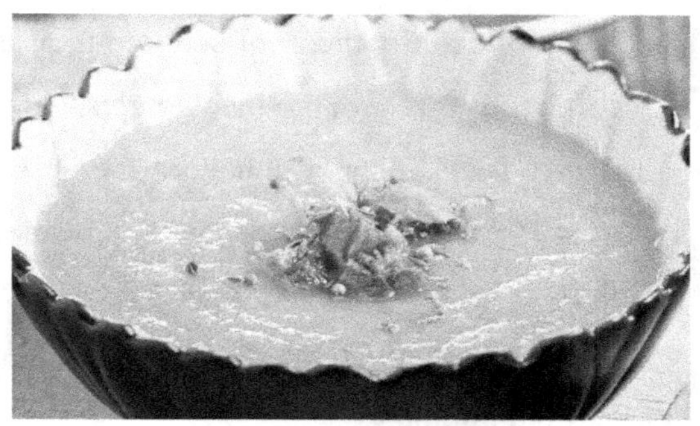

Turmeric Golden Paste

Ingredients:

- 1/2 cup turmeric powder
- 1 cup water
- 1/3 cup coconut oil
- 2-3 teaspoons ground black pepper

Instructions:

1. In a saucepan, combine turmeric powder and water. Stir well to form a smooth paste.

2. Heat the mixture over medium heat, stirring constantly. Continue stirring until you have a thick paste. This typically takes about 7-10 minutes.

3. Once the turmeric paste has thickened, reduce the heat to low and add coconut oil. Stir until the coconut oil is fully incorporated into the paste.

4. Incorporate the ground black pepper into the mixture. Black pepper enhances the absorption of curcumin, the active compound in turmeric.

5. Continue to stir the paste over low heat for an additional 2-3 minutes to ensure all ingredients are well combined.

6. Remove the saucepan from heat and allow the turmeric golden paste to cool.

7. Transfer the cooled paste into a glass jar with a lid.

8. Store the turmeric golden paste in the refrigerator. It can be kept for up to 2 weeks.

Usage:

- Add 1/4 to 1/2 teaspoon of turmeric golden paste to your dishes, smoothies, or beverages.
- Consider using it in recipes for turmeric lattes, curries, soups, or stews.

Garlic and Rosemary Roasted Vegetables

Ingredients:

- 4 cups mixed vegetables (e.g., carrots, potatoes, bell peppers, zucchini, cherry tomatoes), washed and chopped
- 3 tablespoons olive oil
- 4 cloves garlic, minced
- 1 tablespoon fresh rosemary, chopped
- Salt and black pepper to taste

Instructions:

1. Preheat the oven to 425°F (220°C).
2. In a large bowl, combine the chopped mixed vegetables.
3. In a small bowl, mix together olive oil, minced garlic, chopped rosemary, salt, and black pepper.
4. Pour the olive oil mixture over the vegetables and toss until the vegetables are evenly coated.
5. Spread the vegetables in a single layer on a baking sheet lined with parchment paper or a silicone baking mat.

6. Roast in the preheated oven for 25-30 minutes or until the vegetables are golden brown and tender, stirring halfway through to ensure even cooking.

7. Remove the roasted vegetables from the oven and transfer them to a serving dish.

8. Optionally, garnish with additional fresh rosemary for a burst of flavor and visual appeal.

9. Serve the garlic and rosemary roasted vegetables as a delicious side dish for a variety of meals.

Cilantro-Lime Quinoa

Ingredients:

- 1 cup quinoa, rinsed
- 2 cups water or vegetable broth
- 1/4 cup fresh cilantro, chopped
- 1 lime, juiced
- 1 tablespoon olive oil
- Salt and pepper to taste
- Optional: Lime wedges and additional cilantro for garnish

Instructions:

1. Rinse the quinoa under cold water using a fine-mesh sieve to remove any bitterness.

2. In a medium saucepan, combine the rinsed quinoa and water or vegetable broth. Bring to a boil over medium-high heat.

3. Reduce the heat to low, cover, and simmer for 15-20 minutes, or until the quinoa is cooked and the liquid is absorbed. Fluff the quinoa with a fork.

4. In a separate bowl, mix together fresh chopped cilantro, lime juice, olive oil, salt, and pepper.

5. Pour the cilantro-lime mixture over the cooked quinoa.

6. Toss the quinoa gently to ensure it's evenly coated with the cilantro-lime dressing.

7. Taste and adjust the seasoning, adding more salt, pepper, or lime juice as needed.

8. Optional: Garnish with additional cilantro and serve with lime wedges on the side for extra freshness.

9. Serve the cilantro-lime quinoa as a side dish or as a base for other main dishes.

Ginger-Infused Carrot Soup

Ingredients:

- 1 pound carrots, peeled and sliced

- 1 onion, chopped
- 2 cloves garlic, minced
- 1 tablespoon fresh ginger, grated
- 1 tablespoon olive oil
- 4 cups vegetable broth
- 1 teaspoon ground cumin
- 1/2 teaspoon ground coriander
- 1/2 teaspoon turmeric
- Salt and pepper to taste
- 1 cup coconut milk (optional, for creaminess)
- Fresh cilantro or parsley for garnish (optional)

Instructions:

1. In a large pot, heat olive oil over medium heat. Add chopped onions and cook until softened, about 3-4 minutes.

2. Add minced garlic and grated ginger to the pot. Sauté for an additional 1-2 minutes until fragrant.

3. Add sliced carrots to the pot and stir to combine with the onions, garlic, and ginger.

4. Pour in the vegetable broth, ensuring that the carrots are mostly submerged. Bring the mixture to a boil.

5. Reduce the heat to low, cover the pot, and simmer for 20-25 minutes, or until the carrots are tender.

6. Use an immersion blender to blend the soup until smooth. Alternatively, carefully transfer the soup to a blender in batches, blending until smooth, and then return it to the pot.

7. Stir in ground cumin, ground coriander, turmeric, salt, and pepper. Adjust the seasonings to taste.

8. Optional: If you desire creaminess, add coconut milk to the soup and stir until well combined.

9. Allow the soup to simmer for an additional 5-10 minutes to let the flavors meld.

10. Serve the ginger-infused carrot soup hot, garnished with fresh cilantro or parsley if desired.

Basil Pesto with Walnuts

Ingredients:

- 2 cups fresh basil leaves, packed
- 1/2 cup walnuts, toasted
- 1/2 cup freshly grated Parmesan cheese
- 3 cloves garlic, minced

- 1/2 cup extra-virgin olive oil
- 1 tablespoon fresh lemon juice
- Salt and pepper to taste

Instructions:

1. Toast the walnuts in a dry skillet over medium heat for 2-3 minutes, or until fragrant. Be careful not to burn them. Set aside to cool.

2. In a food processor, combine the fresh basil leaves, toasted walnuts, freshly grated Parmesan cheese, and minced garlic.

3. Pulse the ingredients until they are finely chopped and well combined.

4. With the food processor running, gradually stream in the extra-virgin olive oil until the pesto reaches a smooth and creamy consistency.

5. Add fresh lemon juice, salt, and pepper to the pesto. Process briefly to incorporate the additional ingredients.

6. Taste the pesto and adjust the seasonings to your liking. Add more salt, pepper, or lemon juice if needed.

7. If the pesto is too thick, you can add more olive oil in small increments until you achieve the desired consistency.

8. Transfer the basil pesto with walnuts to a jar or airtight container.

9. Store the pesto in the refrigerator. It can be kept for up to a week.

10. Use the basil pesto with walnuts as a flavorful sauce for pasta, a spread for sandwiches, or a topping for grilled meats and vegetables.

Minty Green Tea Smoothie

Ingredients:

- 1 cup brewed green tea, cooled
- 1 banana, frozen
- 1/2 cup fresh spinach leaves
- 1/4 cup fresh mint leaves
- 1/2 cup Greek yogurt
- 1 tablespoon honey (optional, for sweetness)
- Ice cubes (optional, for extra chill)
- Mint leaves for garnish (optional)

Instructions:

1. Brew green tea and let it cool to room temperature or refrigerate for faster cooling.

2. In a blender, combine the cooled green tea, frozen banana, fresh spinach leaves, fresh mint leaves, Greek yogurt, and honey (if using).

3. Optionally, add ice cubes for a colder and thicker smoothie.

4. Blend the ingredients on high speed until smooth and creamy. If the smoothie is too thick, you can add more green tea or water to reach your desired consistency.

5. Taste the smoothie and adjust sweetness by adding more honey if needed.

6. Pour the minty green tea smoothie into a glass.

7. Optionally, garnish with fresh mint leaves for a burst of color and added freshness.

8. Serve immediately and enjoy this refreshing and nutritious minty green tea smoothie!

Thyme and Lemon Grilled Chicken

Ingredients:

- 4 boneless, skinless chicken breasts
- 3 tablespoons olive oil
- 2 tablespoons fresh thyme leaves
- Zest of 1 lemon
- Juice of 1 lemon
- 3 cloves garlic, minced
- 1 teaspoon Dijon mustard
- Salt and black pepper to taste

- Lemon wedges for serving (optional)
- Fresh thyme sprigs for garnish (optional)

Instructions:

1. In a small bowl, whisk together olive oil, fresh thyme leaves, lemon zest, lemon juice, minced garlic, Dijon mustard, salt, and black pepper to create the marinade.

2. Place the chicken breasts in a large, shallow dish or a zip-top plastic bag.

3. Pour the marinade over the chicken, ensuring that each piece is well-coated. If time allows, marinate the chicken in the refrigerator for at least 30 minutes to let the flavors penetrate.

4. Preheat the grill to medium-high heat.

5. Remove the chicken from the marinade, allowing any excess to drip off.

6. Grill the chicken for approximately 6-8 minutes per side or until the internal temperature reaches 165°F (74°C) and the juices run clear. Cooking times may vary depending on the thickness of the chicken breasts.

7. Optional: During the last few minutes of grilling, brush the chicken with any remaining marinade for additional flavor.

8. Once done, transfer the grilled chicken to a serving platter.

9. Optionally, garnish with fresh thyme sprigs and serve with lemon wedges on the side.

10. Serve the thyme and lemon grilled chicken with your favorite side dishes or salads.

Coriander–Lemon Salmon

Ingredients:

- 4 salmon filets
- 2 tablespoons olive oil
- 2 tablespoons fresh coriander (cilantro), chopped
- Zest of 1 lemon
- Juice of 1 lemon
- 2 cloves garlic, minced
- 1 teaspoon ground coriander
- Salt and black pepper to taste
- Lemon wedges for serving (optional)
- Fresh coriander (cilantro) leaves for garnish (optional)

Instructions:

1. Preheat the oven to 400°F (200°C).

2. In a small bowl, mix together olive oil, chopped fresh coriander, lemon zest, lemon juice, minced garlic, ground coriander, salt, and black pepper to create the marinade.

3. Place the salmon filets in a baking dish or on a baking sheet lined with parchment paper.

4. Pour the marinade over the salmon filets, ensuring they are well-coated. You can use a brush to evenly distribute the marinade.

5. Allow the salmon to marinate for at least 15-20 minutes. This gives the flavors time to infuse into the fish.

6. Bake the salmon in the preheated oven for about 12-15 minutes, or until the salmon flakes easily with a fork and is cooked to your desired level of doneness.

7. Optional: During the last few minutes of baking, you can broil the salmon for a slightly crispy top.

8. Once done, remove the salmon from the oven and transfer to a serving platter.

9. Optionally, garnish with fresh coriander leaves and serve with lemon wedges on the side.

10. Serve the coriander-lemon salmon with your favorite side dishes, such as steamed vegetables or rice.

Chamomile-Infused Quinoa Porridge

Ingredients:

- 1 cup quinoa, rinsed
- 2 cups water
- 2 chamomile tea bags
- 2 cups milk (dairy or plant-based)
- 2 tablespoons honey or maple syrup
- 1 teaspoon vanilla extract
- 1/2 teaspoon ground cinnamon
- Pinch of salt
- Optional toppings: Fresh fruits, nuts, seeds, or a drizzle of honey

Instructions:

1. In a saucepan, combine quinoa, water, and chamomile tea bags.
2. Bring the mixture to a boil over medium-high heat, then reduce the heat to low, cover, and simmer for 15 minutes or until the quinoa is cooked and the liquid is absorbed.

3. Remove the tea bags and fluff the quinoa with a fork.

4. In a separate saucepan, heat the milk over medium heat until warm but not boiling.

5. Stir the warm milk into the cooked quinoa.

6. Add honey or maple syrup, vanilla extract, ground cinnamon, and a pinch of salt. Stir well to combine.

7. Simmer the chamomile-infused quinoa porridge over low heat for an additional 5-7 minutes, stirring occasionally, until it reaches your desired consistency.

8. Taste and adjust sweetness if needed, adding more honey or maple syrup.

9. Remove the chamomile-infused quinoa porridge from heat.

10. Serve the porridge in bowls, and top with your favorite fruits, nuts, seeds, or an extra drizzle of honey.

11. Enjoy this soothing and aromatic chamomile-infused quinoa porridge as a comforting breakfast or snack.

Sage and Garlic Buttered Sweet Potatoes

Ingredients:

- 2 large sweet potatoes, peeled and cut into cubes
- 4 tablespoons unsalted butter
- 3 cloves garlic, minced
- 1 tablespoon fresh sage leaves, chopped
- Salt and black pepper to taste
- Optional: 1/4 cup chopped pecans or walnuts (for garnish)
- Optional: Fresh sage leaves for garnish

Instructions:

1. Preheat the oven to 400°F (200°C).
2. In a large pot, bring water to a boil. Add the sweet potato cubes and cook for about 5 minutes or until they are just beginning to soften. Drain and set aside.
3. In a large skillet over medium heat, melt the butter.
4. Add minced garlic to the melted butter and sauté for about 1-2 minutes until fragrant.
5. Add chopped fresh sage leaves to the skillet and continue to sauté for an additional 1-2 minutes.

6. Add the partially cooked sweet potato cubes to the skillet, tossing to coat them evenly with the sage and garlic-infused butter.

7. Season the sweet potatoes with salt and black pepper to taste. Adjust the seasoning if needed.

8. Transfer the sweet potato mixture to a baking dish, spreading it out in an even layer.

9. Bake in the preheated oven for 20-25 minutes or until the sweet potatoes are tender and caramelized around the edges.

10. Optional: In the last 5 minutes of baking, sprinkle chopped pecans or walnuts over the sweet potatoes for added crunch.

11. Once done, remove the sage and garlic buttered sweet potatoes from the oven.

12. Optionally, garnish with fresh sage leaves for a decorative touch.

13. Serve the sweet potatoes as a delicious and savory side dish.

Rosemary Citrus Fruit Salad

Ingredients:

- 2 cups mixed citrus fruits (oranges, grapefruits, mandarins), peeled and segmented

- 1 cup strawberries, hulled and sliced
- 1 cup pineapple chunks
- 1 tablespoon fresh rosemary, finely chopped
- 2 tablespoons honey
- 1 tablespoon fresh orange juice
- 1 teaspoon lemon zest
- Optional: Mint leaves for garnish

Instructions:

1. In a large bowl, combine the mixed citrus fruits, sliced strawberries, and pineapple chunks.
2. In a small bowl, whisk together the honey, fresh orange juice, and lemon zest.
3. Pour the honey and citrus dressing over the fruit mixture.
4. Add the finely chopped fresh rosemary to the bowl.
5. Gently toss the fruit salad until all the ingredients are well coated with the dressing.
6. Allow the rosemary citrus fruit salad to marinate for at least 15 minutes to let the flavors meld.
7. Optional: Garnish the fruit salad with fresh mint leaves for a burst of color and added freshness.
8. Serve the rosemary citrus fruit salad chilled as a refreshing and aromatic side dish or dessert.

Dill and Yogurt Cucumber Salad

Ingredients:

- 3 large cucumbers, thinly sliced
- 1 cup plain Greek yogurt
- 2 tablespoons fresh dill, chopped
- 1 clove garlic, minced
- 1 tablespoon extra-virgin olive oil
- 1 tablespoon white wine vinegar
- Salt and black pepper to taste

Instructions:

1. In a large bowl, combine the thinly sliced cucumbers.
2. In a separate bowl, whisk together Greek yogurt, chopped fresh dill, minced garlic, olive oil, and white wine vinegar.
3. Pour the yogurt and dill dressing over the sliced cucumbers.
4. Toss the cucumber slices until they are well coated with the dill and yogurt dressing.
5. Season the cucumber salad with salt and black pepper to taste. Adjust the seasoning if needed.

6. Allow the cucumber salad to chill in the refrigerator for at least 30 minutes before serving. This helps the flavors meld and enhances the crispness of the cucumbers.

7. Before serving, give the salad a final gentle toss to redistribute the dressing.

8. Optionally, garnish with extra dill leaves for added freshness.

9. Serve the dill and yogurt cucumber salad as a cool and refreshing side dish.

Oregano and Tomato Quinoa Salad

Ingredients:

- 1 cup quinoa, rinsed
- 2 cups water
- 1 cup cherry tomatoes, halved
- 1 cucumber, diced
- 1/2 red onion, finely chopped
- 1/4 cup Kalamata olives, sliced
- 1/4 cup feta cheese, crumbled
- 2 tablespoons fresh oregano leaves, chopped
- 3 tablespoons extra-virgin olive oil
- 1 tablespoon red wine vinegar
- Salt and black pepper to taste

- Optional: Lemon wedges for serving

Instructions:

1. In a medium saucepan, combine quinoa and water. Bring to a boil, then reduce heat to low, cover, and simmer for 15-20 minutes or until quinoa is cooked and water is absorbed.
2. Fluff the quinoa with a fork and let it cool to room temperature.
3. In a large bowl, combine the cooked quinoa, cherry tomatoes, diced cucumber, chopped red onion, sliced Kalamata olives, crumbled feta cheese, and chopped fresh oregano.
4. In a small bowl, whisk together extra-virgin olive oil, red wine vinegar, salt, and black pepper.
5. Pour the dressing over the quinoa and vegetable mixture. Toss gently to combine, ensuring everything is well coated with the dressing.
6. Taste the quinoa salad and adjust the seasoning if needed.
7. Allow the salad to sit in the refrigerator for at least 30 minutes before serving. This helps the flavors meld and enhances the overall taste.

8. Optionally, garnish the oregano and tomato quinoa salad with additional fresh oregano leaves.

9. Serve the salad chilled as a delicious and nutritious side dish or a light meal.

"I am grateful for the abundance of fresh, natural foods that fuel my body's resilience."

"Choosing nutrient-rich options aligns with my goal of fostering a strong and vibrant body."

CHAPTER 8: SALADS AND DESSERTS

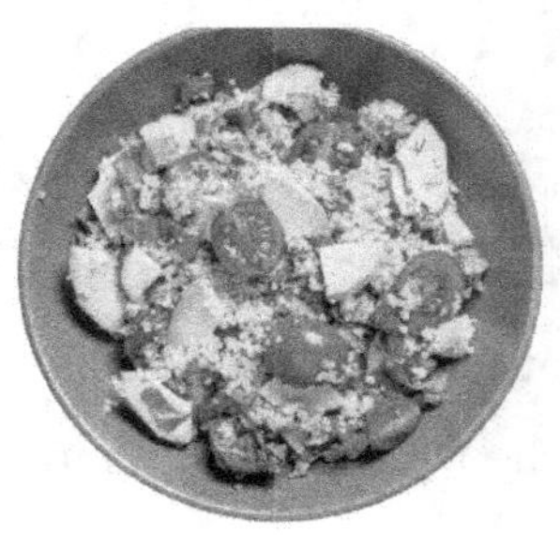

SALADS

Kale and Berry Salad

Ingredients:

For the Salad:

- 4 cups kale, stems removed and leaves chopped
- 1 cup mixed berries (strawberries, blueberries, raspberries, etc.)
- 1/2 cup feta cheese, crumbled
- 1/4 cup red onion, thinly sliced
- 1/4 cup sliced almonds, toasted

For the Dressing:

- 3 tablespoons extra-virgin olive oil

- 2 tablespoons balsamic vinegar
- 1 tablespoon honey
- 1 teaspoon Dijon mustard
- Salt and black pepper to taste

Instructions:

1. In a large bowl, place the chopped kale.
2. In a small bowl, whisk together the dressing ingredients: extra-virgin olive oil, balsamic vinegar, honey, Dijon mustard, salt, and black pepper.
3. Pour the dressing over the kale and massage it into the leaves. This helps to tenderize the kale and allows it to absorb the flavors.
4. Let the kale sit for about 10-15 minutes to marinate.
5. Add the mixed berries, crumbled feta cheese, thinly sliced red onion, and toasted sliced almonds to the kale.
6. Toss all the ingredients together until the salad is well combined and evenly coated with the dressing.
7. Taste the salad and adjust the seasoning if needed.

8. Optionally, garnish with additional feta cheese or almonds.

9. Serve the kale and berry salad immediately as a vibrant and refreshing side dish or a light meal.

Quinoa Spinach Salad with Citrus Dressing

Ingredients:

For the Salad:

- 1 cup quinoa, rinsed
- 2 cups water
- 4 cups fresh spinach leaves, washed and chopped
- 1 cup cherry tomatoes, halved
- 1 cucumber, diced
- 1/4 cup red onion, finely chopped
- 1/3 cup feta cheese, crumbled
- 1/4 cup pine nuts, toasted

For the Citrus Dressing:

- Juice of 2 oranges
- Juice of 1 lemon
- 3 tablespoons extra-virgin olive oil
- 1 teaspoon Dijon mustard
- 1 tablespoon honey

- Salt and black pepper to taste

Instructions:

1. In a medium saucepan, combine quinoa and water. Bring to a boil, then reduce heat to low, cover, and simmer for 15-20 minutes or until quinoa is cooked and water is absorbed.
2. Fluff the quinoa with a fork and let it cool to room temperature.
3. In a large bowl, combine the cooked quinoa, chopped fresh spinach, cherry tomatoes, diced cucumber, chopped red onion, crumbled feta cheese, and toasted pine nuts.
4. In a small bowl, whisk together the dressing ingredients: orange juice, lemon juice, extra-virgin olive oil, Dijon mustard, honey, salt, and black pepper.
5. Pour the citrus dressing over the quinoa and vegetable mixture. Toss gently to combine, ensuring everything is well coated with the dressing.
6. Taste the quinoa salad and adjust the seasoning if needed.

7. Allow the salad to sit in the refrigerator for at least 30 minutes before serving. This helps the flavors meld and enhances the overall taste.

8. Optionally, garnish the quinoa spinach salad with additional feta cheese or pine nuts.

9. Serve the salad chilled as a nutritious and flavorful side dish or a light meal.

Turmeric Chickpea Salad

Ingredients:

For the Turmeric Chickpeas:

- 2 cans (15 ounces each) chickpeas, drained and rinsed
- 2 tablespoons olive oil
- 1 teaspoon ground turmeric
- 1/2 teaspoon ground cumin
- 1/2 teaspoon smoked paprika
- Salt and black pepper to taste

For the Salad:

- 4 cups mixed salad greens (e.g., spinach, arugula, kale)
- 1 cucumber, diced
- 1 cup cherry tomatoes, halved
- 1/4 cup red onion, thinly sliced

- 1/4 cup fresh cilantro, chopped

For the Turmeric Tahini Dressing:

- 1/4 cup tahini
- 2 tablespoons olive oil
- 1 tablespoon apple cider vinegar
- 1 tablespoon lemon juice
- 1 teaspoon ground turmeric
- 1 teaspoon honey
- Salt and black pepper to taste
- Water (as needed to thin the dressing)

Instructions:

For the Turmeric Chickpeas:

1. Preheat the oven to 400°F (200°C).
2. In a bowl, toss the drained and rinsed chickpeas with olive oil, ground turmeric, ground cumin, smoked paprika, salt, and black pepper.
3. Spread the seasoned chickpeas on a baking sheet in a single layer.
4. Roast in the preheated oven for 25-30 minutes or until the chickpeas are golden and crispy, shaking the pan occasionally for even cooking.
5. Remove from the oven and let the turmeric chickpeas cool slightly.

For the Salad:

6. In a large salad bowl, combine the mixed greens, diced cucumber, cherry tomatoes, sliced red onion, and chopped fresh cilantro.

7. Add the roasted turmeric chickpeas to the salad.

For the Turmeric Tahini Dressing:

8. In a small bowl, whisk together tahini, olive oil, apple cider vinegar, lemon juice, ground turmeric, honey, salt, and black pepper.

9. If the dressing is too thick, add water a tablespoon at a time until it reaches your desired consistency.

10. Drizzle the turmeric tahini dressing over the salad and toss gently to coat.

11. Taste the salad and adjust the seasoning or add more dressing if needed.

12. Serve the turmeric chickpea salad immediately, enjoying the vibrant colors and flavors.

Broccoli and Almond Salad

Ingredients:

- 4 cups broccoli florets, blanched and cooled
- 1/2 cup sliced almonds, toasted
- 1/4 cup red onion, finely chopped

- 1/4 cup dried cranberries or raisins
- 1/3 cup feta cheese, crumbled

For the Lemon Poppy Seed Dressing:

- 1/4 cup olive oil
- 2 tablespoons lemon juice
- 1 tablespoon honey
- 1 teaspoon Dijon mustard
- 1 teaspoon poppy seeds
- Salt and black pepper to taste

Instructions:

For the Lemon Poppy Seed Dressing:

1. In a small bowl, whisk together olive oil, lemon juice, honey, Dijon mustard, poppy seeds, salt, and black pepper.

2. Set aside the dressing to allow the flavors to meld.

For the Broccoli and Almond Salad:

3. Blanch the broccoli florets in boiling water for 2-3 minutes or until they are bright green. Immediately transfer them to an ice bath to stop the cooking process. Once cooled, drain and pat dry.

4. In a large salad bowl, combine the blanched broccoli florets, toasted sliced almonds, finely chopped red onion, dried cranberries or raisins, and crumbled feta cheese.

5. Drizzle the lemon poppy seed dressing over the salad.

6. Gently toss the salad to ensure all ingredients are well coated with the dressing.

7. Allow the broccoli and almond salad to sit for a few minutes to absorb the flavors.

8. Taste and adjust the seasoning, adding more salt or pepper if needed.

9. Serve the salad immediately as a refreshing and crunchy side dish.

Cabbage and Carrot Slaw with Ginger Dressing

Ingredients:

For the Cabbage and Carrot Slaw:

- 4 cups green cabbage, finely shredded
- 2 cups carrots, julienned or grated
- 1/2 cup red cabbage, finely shredded (optional, for color)
- 1/4 cup green onions, thinly sliced

- 1/4 cup cilantro, chopped (optional, for added freshness)
- 1/4 cup sesame seeds, toasted (optional, for garnish)

For the Ginger Dressing:

- 3 tablespoons rice vinegar
- 2 tablespoons soy sauce
- 1 tablespoon sesame oil
- 1 tablespoon fresh ginger, grated
- 1 tablespoon honey or maple syrup
- 1 clove garlic, minced
- 1/4 cup neutral oil (vegetable or grapeseed)
- Salt and black pepper to taste

Instructions:

For the Cabbage and Carrot Slaw:

1. In a large bowl, combine the finely shredded green cabbage, julienned or grated carrots, optional finely shredded red cabbage, sliced green onions, and chopped cilantro.
2. Toss the ingredients together until they are evenly distributed.
3. If using, sprinkle toasted sesame seeds over the slaw for a nutty crunch.

For the Ginger Dressing:

4. In a small bowl, whisk together rice vinegar, soy sauce, sesame oil, grated fresh ginger, honey or maple syrup, minced garlic, neutral oil, salt, and black pepper.

5. Taste the dressing and adjust the sweetness or saltiness according to your preference.

6. Pour the ginger dressing over the cabbage and carrot slaw.

7. Toss the slaw and dressing together until all ingredients are well coated.

8. Allow the slaw to sit for a few minutes to let the flavors meld.

9. Optionally, garnish with additional cilantro or sesame seeds before serving.

10. Serve the cabbage and carrot slaw with ginger dressing immediately as a crisp and flavorful side dish.

Beet and Walnut Salad with Goat Cheese

Ingredients:

For the Beet and Walnut Salad:

- 4 medium beets, roasted, peeled, and diced

- 1 cup arugula or mixed salad greens
- 1/2 cup walnuts, toasted and chopped
- 1/4 cup red onion, thinly sliced
- 1/3 cup crumbled goat cheese
- Fresh parsley, chopped (for garnish)

For the Balsamic Vinaigrette:

- 3 tablespoons balsamic vinegar
- 2 tablespoons extra-virgin olive oil
- 1 teaspoon Dijon mustard
- 1 teaspoon honey
- Salt and black pepper to taste

Instructions:

For the Beet and Walnut Salad:

1. Preheat the oven to 400°F (200°C).
2. Wash and trim the beets, leaving the skin on. Wrap each beet in aluminum foil and place them on a baking sheet.
3. Roast the beets in the preheated oven for about 45-60 minutes or until they are tender. Allow them to cool, then peel and dice.
4. In a large salad bowl, combine the diced roasted beets, arugula or mixed salad greens, toasted and chopped walnuts, thinly sliced red onion, and crumbled goat cheese.

5. Toss the salad ingredients together until well combined.

For the Balsamic Vinaigrette:

6. In a small bowl, whisk together balsamic vinegar, extra-virgin olive oil, Dijon mustard, honey, salt, and black pepper.

7. Taste the vinaigrette and adjust the sweetness or acidity according to your preference.

8. Drizzle the balsamic vinaigrette over the beet and walnut salad.

9. Gently toss the salad to ensure all ingredients are well coated with the dressing.

10. Allow the salad to sit for a few minutes to let the flavors meld.

11. Garnish the salad with chopped fresh parsley.

12. Serve the beet and walnut salad with goat cheese immediately as a colorful and flavorful side dish.

Avocado, Tomato, and Chickpea Salad

Ingredients:

- 1 can (15 ounces) chickpeas, drained and rinsed
- 2 ripe avocados, diced
- 1 pint cherry tomatoes, halved

- 1/4 cup red onion, finely chopped
- 1/4 cup fresh cilantro, chopped
- 1/4 cup feta cheese, crumbled (optional)

For the Dressing:

- 3 tablespoons extra-virgin olive oil
- 2 tablespoons balsamic vinegar
- 1 teaspoon Dijon mustard
- 1 clove garlic, minced
- Salt and black pepper to taste

Instructions:

1. In a large bowl, combine the drained and rinsed chickpeas, diced avocados, halved cherry tomatoes, chopped red onion, and chopped fresh cilantro.
2. If using, add crumbled feta cheese to the salad ingredients.
3. In a small bowl, whisk together the dressing ingredients: extra-virgin olive oil, balsamic vinegar, Dijon mustard, minced garlic, salt, and black pepper.
4. Pour the dressing over the chickpea salad.
5. Gently toss the salad to ensure all ingredients are well coated with the dressing.

6. Taste the salad and adjust the seasoning if needed.

7. Allow the salad to sit for a few minutes to let the flavors meld.

8. Serve the avocado, tomato, and chickpea salad immediately as a refreshing and nutrient-packed side dish or light meal.

Arugula and Pomegranate Salad

Ingredients:

- 4 cups arugula, washed and dried
- 1 cup pomegranate arils (seeds)
- 1/2 cup crumbled feta cheese
- 1/4 cup red onion, thinly sliced
- 1/3 cup toasted pecans or walnuts, chopped

For the Lemon Vinaigrette:

- 3 tablespoons extra-virgin olive oil
- 2 tablespoons lemon juice
- 1 teaspoon Dijon mustard
- 1 teaspoon honey
- Salt and black pepper to taste

Instructions:

1. In a large salad bowl, combine the arugula, pomegranate arils, crumbled feta cheese, thinly sliced red onion, and toasted nuts.

2. In a small bowl, whisk together the lemon vinaigrette ingredients: extra-virgin olive oil, lemon juice, Dijon mustard, honey, salt, and black pepper.

3. Pour the lemon vinaigrette over the salad.

4. Gently toss the salad to ensure all ingredients are well coated with the dressing.

5. Taste the salad and adjust the seasoning if needed.

6. Allow the arugula and pomegranate salad to sit for a few minutes to let the flavors meld.

7. Serve the salad immediately as a vibrant and refreshing side dish or light meal.

Orange and Fennel Quinoa Salad

Ingredients:

For the Orange and Fennel Quinoa Salad:

- 1 cup quinoa, rinsed
- 2 cups water
- 2 medium oranges, peeled and segmented

- 1 medium fennel bulb, thinly sliced
- 1/4 cup red onion, finely chopped
- 1/3 cup fresh parsley, chopped
- 1/4 cup sliced almonds, toasted
- Salt and black pepper to taste

For the Orange Vinaigrette:

- Juice of 1 orange
- 2 tablespoons extra-virgin olive oil
- 1 tablespoon white wine vinegar
- 1 teaspoon honey
- 1/2 teaspoon Dijon mustard
- Salt and black pepper to taste

Instructions:

For the Orange and Fennel Quinoa Salad:

1. In a medium saucepan, combine quinoa and water. Bring to a boil, then reduce heat to low, cover, and simmer for 15-20 minutes or until quinoa is cooked and water is absorbed.

2. Fluff the quinoa with a fork and let it cool to room temperature.

3. In a large bowl, combine the cooked quinoa, orange segments, thinly sliced fennel, finely chopped red onion, chopped fresh parsley, and toasted sliced almonds.

4. Season the salad with salt and black pepper to taste. Toss the ingredients together until well combined.

For the Orange Vinaigrette:

5. In a small bowl, whisk together the orange juice, extra-virgin olive oil, white wine vinegar, honey, Dijon mustard, salt, and black pepper.

6. Pour the orange vinaigrette over the quinoa salad.

7. Gently toss the salad to ensure all ingredients are well coated with the dressing.

8. Taste the salad and adjust the seasoning if needed.

9. Allow the salad to sit for a few minutes to let the flavors meld.

10. Serve the orange and fennel quinoa salad immediately as a vibrant and flavorful side dish or light meal.

Mango Cucumber Salsa Salad

Ingredients:

- 2 ripe mangoes, peeled, pitted, and diced
- 1 cucumber, peeled and diced
- 1/2 red onion, finely chopped

- 1 red bell pepper, diced
- 1 jalapeño, seeds removed and finely chopped (optional, for heat)
- 1/4 cup fresh cilantro, chopped
- Juice of 2 limes
- Salt and black pepper to taste
- Tortilla chips or crackers (for serving)

Instructions:

1. In a large bowl, combine the diced mangoes, diced cucumber, finely chopped red onion, diced red bell pepper, chopped jalapeño (if using), and chopped fresh cilantro.
2. Squeeze the juice of two limes over the ingredients in the bowl.
3. Season the mango cucumber salsa salad with salt and black pepper to taste.
4. Gently toss the ingredients together until well combined.
5. Taste the salsa and adjust the seasoning or add more lime juice if needed.
6. Allow the mango cucumber salsa salad to sit for a few minutes to let the flavors meld.
7. Serve the salsa salad in a bowl alongside tortilla chips or crackers.

8. Enjoy this vibrant and refreshing mango cucumber salsa salad as a delicious appetizer or a light and fruity side dish.

Tomato Basil Mozzarella Salad

Ingredients:

- 4 cups cherry tomatoes, halved
- 1 cup fresh mozzarella balls (bocconcini), halved
- 1/2 cup fresh basil leaves, torn
- 2 tablespoons extra-virgin olive oil
- 1 tablespoon balsamic glaze
- Salt and black pepper to taste

Instructions:

1. In a large bowl, combine the halved cherry tomatoes, halved mozzarella balls, and torn fresh basil leaves.
2. Drizzle the extra-virgin olive oil over the tomato, basil, and mozzarella mixture.
3. Drizzle the balsamic glaze over the salad for a sweet and tangy flavor.
4. Season the salad with salt and black pepper to taste.

5. Gently toss the ingredients together until well combined and evenly coated with the olive oil and balsamic glaze.

6. Taste the tomato basil mozzarella salad and adjust the seasoning if needed.

7. Allow the salad to sit for a few minutes to let the flavors meld.

8. Serve the salad in a shallow dish or on a platter.

9. Optionally, garnish with additional fresh basil leaves for a decorative touch.

10. Enjoy this classic and refreshing tomato basil mozzarella salad as a light and flavorful appetizer or side dish.

Lentil and Vegetable Salad

Ingredients:

For the Lentils:

- 1 cup dried green or brown lentils
- 3 cups water
- 1 bay leaf
- 1 clove garlic, minced
- Salt to taste

For the Salad:

- 2 cups cherry tomatoes, halved

- 1 cucumber, diced
- 1 red bell pepper, diced
- 1/2 red onion, finely chopped
- 1/3 cup fresh parsley, chopped

For the Dressing:

- 3 tablespoons extra-virgin olive oil
- 2 tablespoons red wine vinegar
- 1 teaspoon Dijon mustard
- 1 clove garlic, minced
- Salt and black pepper to taste

Instructions:

For the Lentils:

1. Rinse the lentils under cold water.
2. In a medium saucepan, combine the rinsed lentils, water, bay leaf, minced garlic, and a pinch of salt.
3. Bring the water to a boil, then reduce the heat to low, cover, and simmer for about 20-25 minutes or until the lentils are tender but still hold their shape.
4. Drain any excess water and remove the bay leaf.
5. Let the lentils cool to room temperature.

For the Salad:

6. In a large bowl, combine the cooked lentils, halved cherry tomatoes, diced cucumber, diced red bell pepper, finely chopped red onion, and chopped fresh parsley.

For the Dressing:

7. In a small bowl, whisk together the extra-virgin olive oil, red wine vinegar, Dijon mustard, minced garlic, salt, and black pepper.
8. Pour the dressing over the lentil and vegetable mixture.
9. Gently toss the salad to ensure all ingredients are well coated with the dressing.
10. Taste the lentil and vegetable salad and adjust the seasoning if needed.
11. Allow the salad to sit for a few minutes to let the flavors meld.
12. Serve the lentil and vegetable salad at room temperature or chilled.

Mixed Berry Chia Seed Pudding

Ingredients:

For the Chia Seed Pudding:

- 1/2 cup chia seeds
- 2 cups almond milk (or any milk of your choice)
- 2 tablespoons maple syrup or honey
- 1 teaspoon vanilla extract

For the Mixed Berry Compote:

- 1 cup mixed berries (strawberries, blueberries, raspberries)
- 2 tablespoons maple syrup or honey
- 1 tablespoon lemon juice
- 1 teaspoon cornstarch mixed with 1 tablespoon water (optional, for thickening)

For Assembly:

- Fresh mixed berries for topping
- Granola for crunch (optional)

Instructions:

For the Chia Seed Pudding:

1. In a bowl, combine chia seeds, almond milk, maple syrup or honey, and vanilla extract.

2. Whisk the ingredients together until well combined.

3. Let the chia seed mixture sit for 5-10 minutes, then whisk again to prevent clumping.

4. Cover the bowl and refrigerate for at least 3 hours or overnight to allow the chia seeds to absorb the liquid and create a pudding-like consistency.

For the Mixed Berry Compote:

5. In a saucepan, combine mixed berries, maple syrup or honey, and lemon juice.

6. Cook over medium heat, stirring occasionally, until the berries break down and the mixture thickens slightly.

7. If you prefer a thicker compote, mix cornstarch with water to create a slurry and add it to the berry mixture. Stir well and cook for an additional 2-3 minutes.

8. Remove the berry compote from heat and let it cool to room temperature.

For Assembly:

9. Once the chia seed pudding has set, give it a good stir to ensure a smooth texture.

10. Spoon the chia seed pudding into serving glasses or bowls.

11. Top the pudding with the mixed berry compote.

12. Garnish with fresh mixed berries and granola if desired.

13. Serve the mixed berry chia seed pudding immediately or refrigerate until ready to serve.

Turmeric Mango Sorbet

Ingredients:

- 3 cups ripe mango, peeled and diced
- 1 cup coconut milk
- 1/2 cup sugar (adjust according to sweetness preference)
- 1 teaspoon turmeric powder
- 1 tablespoon lime or lemon juice
- Pinch of black pepper (optional, enhances turmeric absorption)
- Pinch of salt

Instructions:

1. Peel and dice ripe mangoes, ensuring you have about 3 cups of mango chunks.

2. In a blender, combine the diced mango, coconut milk, sugar, turmeric powder, lime or lemon juice, black pepper (if using), and a pinch of salt.

3. Blend the ingredients until you achieve a smooth and creamy consistency.

4. Taste the mixture and adjust the sweetness or acidity by adding more sugar or lime/lemon juice if needed.

5. Once satisfied with the taste, pour the mango mixture into a bowl or container suitable for freezing.

6. Cover the container with a lid or plastic wrap and place it in the freezer.

7. After about 1-2 hours, take the container out and stir the mixture to break up any ice crystals that may have formed.

8. Repeat this process every 1-2 hours for the next 4-6 hours, or until the sorbet reaches the desired consistency.

9. Once the turmeric mango sorbet has a smooth and scoopable texture, let it freeze for an additional 2-4 hours or overnight for the best results.

10. Before serving, let the sorbet sit at room temperature for a few minutes to soften slightly.

11. Scoop the turmeric mango sorbet into bowls or cones, and enjoy this refreshing and tropical treat!

Dark Chocolate Avocado Mousse

Ingredients:

- 2 ripe avocados, peeled and pitted
- 1/2 cup dark chocolate chips or chopped dark chocolate (70% cocoa or higher)
- 1/4 cup unsweetened cocoa powder
- 1/4 cup maple syrup or honey (adjust to taste)
- 1 teaspoon vanilla extract
- Pinch of salt
- Optional toppings: whipped cream, berries, chopped nuts

Instructions:

1. In a microwave-safe bowl, melt the dark chocolate chips or chopped dark chocolate. Heat in 20-second intervals, stirring between each interval, until fully melted. Alternatively, you can melt the chocolate using a double boiler on the stove.

2. In a blender or food processor, combine the ripe avocados, melted dark chocolate, cocoa powder, maple syrup or honey, vanilla extract, and a pinch of salt.

3. Blend the ingredients until you achieve a smooth and creamy consistency, scraping down the sides as needed to ensure even blending.

4. Taste the dark chocolate avocado mousse and adjust the sweetness or cocoa intensity by adding more maple syrup or cocoa powder if desired.

5. Once the mousse reaches a satisfying taste and texture, transfer it to serving bowls or glasses.

6. Cover the bowls or glasses with plastic wrap, ensuring the wrap touches the surface of the mousse to prevent oxidation.

7. Refrigerate the dark chocolate avocado mousse for at least 2 hours to chill and allow the flavors to meld.

8. Before serving, let the mousse sit at room temperature for a few minutes to soften slightly.

9. Optionally, garnish the mousse with whipped cream, berries, or chopped nuts.

10. Serve this decadent dark chocolate avocado mousse as a rich and creamy dessert.

Baked Apples with Cinnamon and Walnuts

Ingredients:

- 4 medium-sized apples (such as Granny Smith or Honeycrisp)
- 1/4 cup chopped walnuts
- 2 tablespoons brown sugar
- 1 teaspoon ground cinnamon
- 2 tablespoons unsalted butter, melted
- 1/2 cup apple cider or apple juice
- Vanilla ice cream or whipped cream for serving (optional)

Instructions:

1. Preheat your oven to 375°F (190°C).
2. Wash and core the apples, leaving the bottom intact to create a well for the filling.
3. In a small bowl, mix together the chopped walnuts, brown sugar, and ground cinnamon.
4. Place the cored apples in a baking dish.
5. Stuff each apple with the walnut mixture, pressing it down gently.

6. Drizzle melted butter over the top of each stuffed apple.

7. Pour apple cider or apple juice into the bottom of the baking dish.

8. Bake in the preheated oven for 30-40 minutes or until the apples are tender but not mushy. Baking time may vary depending on the size and type of apples.

9. Occasionally, spoon some of the liquid from the baking dish over the apples to keep them moist.

10. Once baked, remove the apples from the oven and let them cool for a few minutes.

11. Serve the baked apples warm, optionally topped with a scoop of vanilla ice cream or a dollop of whipped cream.

12. Drizzle any remaining juices from the baking dish over the apples before serving.

Quinoa and Almond Flour Cookies

Ingredients:

- 1 cup cooked quinoa, cooled
- 1 cup almond flour
- 1/2 cup coconut oil, melted
- 1/2 cup maple syrup or honey

- 1 teaspoon vanilla extract
- 1/2 teaspoon baking powder
- 1/4 teaspoon salt
- 1/2 cup chocolate chips or chopped nuts (optional)

Instructions:

1. Preheat your oven to 350°F (175°C) and line a baking sheet with parchment paper.

2. In a large mixing bowl, combine the cooked quinoa, almond flour, melted coconut oil, maple syrup or honey, vanilla extract, baking powder, and salt.

3. Mix the ingredients together until well combined.

4. If desired, fold in chocolate chips or chopped nuts to add texture and flavor to the cookies.

5. Using a tablespoon or cookie scoop, drop portions of the cookie dough onto the prepared baking sheet, leaving some space between each cookie.

6. Flatten each cookie slightly with the back of the spoon or your fingers, as these cookies won't spread much during baking.

7. Bake in the preheated oven for 10-12 minutes or until the edges are golden brown.

8. Allow the quinoa and almond flour cookies to cool on the baking sheet for a few minutes before transferring them to a wire rack to cool completely.

9. Once cooled, store the cookies in an airtight container at room temperature.

10. Enjoy these nutritious quinoa and almond flour cookies as a wholesome and gluten-free treat!

Berry and Yogurt Parfait

Ingredients:

- 1 cup Greek yogurt (vanilla or plain)
- 2 tablespoons honey or maple syrup
- 1 cup mixed berries (strawberries, blueberries, raspberries)
- 1/2 cup granola
- 2 tablespoons sliced almonds or chopped nuts
- Fresh mint leaves for garnish (optional)

Instructions:

1. In a bowl, mix Greek yogurt with honey or maple syrup until well combined. Adjust sweetness to your liking.

2. Rinse the mixed berries and pat them dry with a paper towel.

3. In serving glasses or bowls, layer the berry and yogurt parfait. Start with a spoonful of the sweetened Greek yogurt.

4. Add a layer of mixed berries on top of the yogurt.

5. Sprinkle a layer of granola over the berries.

6. Repeat the layers until you reach the top of the glass or bowl, finishing with a layer of berries.

7. Top the parfait with sliced almonds or chopped nuts for added crunch.

8. Optionally, garnish with fresh mint leaves for a burst of freshness.

9. Serve the berry and yogurt parfait immediately as a wholesome and delicious breakfast, snack, or dessert.

Pumpkin Spice Energy Bites

Ingredients:

- 1 cup rolled oats
- 1/2 cup pumpkin puree
- 1/4 cup almond butter (or any nut/seed butter)
- 1/4 cup honey or maple syrup

- 1/3 cup ground flaxseed
- 1/2 teaspoon pumpkin pie spice
- 1/2 teaspoon vanilla extract
- Pinch of salt
- Optional: 1/4 cup chopped nuts, seeds, or mini chocolate chips for added texture

Instructions:

1. In a large mixing bowl, combine rolled oats, pumpkin puree, almond butter, honey or maple syrup, ground flaxseed, pumpkin pie spice, vanilla extract, and a pinch of salt.

2. If desired, fold in chopped nuts, seeds, or mini chocolate chips for added texture and flavor.

3. Mix the ingredients until well combined. The mixture should be sticky and easy to form into balls.

4. Place the bowl in the refrigerator for 15-30 minutes to firm up the mixture, making it easier to shape.

5. Once the mixture has chilled, use your hands to scoop out small portions and roll them into bite-sized energy balls.

6. Arrange the pumpkin spice energy bites on a parchment-lined tray or plate.

7. Refrigerate the energy bites for at least 1 hour to allow them to set and firm up.

8. Once set, transfer the energy bites to an airtight container and store them in the refrigerator.

9. Enjoy these pumpkin spice energy bites as a quick and nutritious snack or energy boost!

Coconut Matcha Popsicles

Ingredients:

- 1 can (14 ounces) coconut milk (full-fat)
- 2 teaspoons matcha powder
- 1/4 cup honey or maple syrup (adjust to taste)
- 1 teaspoon vanilla extract
- Optional: Shredded coconut or chopped pistachios for garnish

Instructions:

1. In a blender, combine coconut milk, matcha powder, honey or maple syrup, and vanilla extract.

2. Blend the ingredients until smooth and well combined. Taste the mixture and adjust sweetness if needed.

3. Optionally, fold in shredded coconut or chopped pistachios for added texture.

4. Pour the matcha coconut mixture into popsicle molds, leaving a little space at the top for expansion.

5. Insert popsicle sticks into the molds.

6. Place the popsicle molds in the freezer and let them freeze for at least 4-6 hours or until completely solid.

7. Once the coconut matcha popsicles are frozen, run the molds under warm water for a few seconds to loosen the popsicles.

8. Gently remove the popsicles from the molds.

9. Optionally, roll the edges of the popsicles in shredded coconut or chopped pistachios for a decorative touch.

10. Serve and enjoy these refreshing and creamy coconut matcha popsicles!

Cinnamon-Spiced Baked Pears

Ingredients:

- 4 ripe but firm pears (such as Bosc or Anjou)
- 2 tablespoons unsalted butter, melted
- 1/4 cup brown sugar
- 1 teaspoon ground cinnamon
- 1/4 teaspoon ground nutmeg

- Pinch of salt

- 1/4 cup chopped nuts (walnuts or pecans), optional

- Vanilla ice cream or Greek yogurt for serving, optional

Instructions:

1. Preheat your oven to 375°F (190°C).

2. Wash and halve the pears. Core them and remove the seeds, creating a hollow in the center.

3. Place the pear halves in a baking dish, cut side up.

4. In a small bowl, mix melted butter, brown sugar, ground cinnamon, ground nutmeg, and a pinch of salt.

5. Spoon the cinnamon-spiced mixture over each pear half, ensuring they are well coated.

6. If desired, sprinkle chopped nuts over the top of the pears.

7. Bake in the preheated oven for about 25-30 minutes or until the pears are tender when pierced with a fork.

8. Optionally, during baking, baste the pears with the juices in the baking dish to enhance the flavor.

9. Once baked, remove the cinnamon-spiced baked pears from the oven and let them cool for a few minutes.

10. Serve the baked pears warm, optionally with a scoop of vanilla ice cream or a dollop of Greek yogurt.

11. Drizzle any remaining juices from the baking dish over the pears before serving.

Oat and Date Bars

Ingredients:

For the Oat and Date Base:

- 1 cup old-fashioned rolled oats
- 1 cup all-purpose flour
- 1/2 cup unsalted butter, softened
- 1/2 cup brown sugar, packed
- 1/4 teaspoon baking soda
- 1/4 teaspoon salt

For the Date Filling:

- 2 cups Medjool dates, pitted and chopped
- 1/2 cup water

- 1 tablespoon lemon juice
- 1/2 teaspoon vanilla extract

For the Oat Crumble Topping:

- 1/2 cup old-fashioned rolled oats
- 2 tablespoons unsalted butter, melted
- 1 tablespoon brown sugar

Instructions:

1. Preheat your oven to 350°F (175°C). Grease or line a square baking pan (8x8 inches or similar) with parchment paper.

2. In a large mixing bowl, combine the rolled oats, all-purpose flour, softened butter, brown sugar, baking soda, and salt for the oat and date base. Mix until the ingredients come together and form a crumbly texture.

3. Press about two-thirds of the oat mixture into the bottom of the prepared baking pan to create an even base.

4. In a saucepan, combine the chopped dates, water, lemon juice, and vanilla extract for the date filling. Cook over medium heat, stirring frequently, until the dates soften and the mixture thickens into a cohesive filling.

5. Spread the date filling evenly over the oat base in the baking pan.

6. In a small bowl, mix the remaining rolled oats, melted butter, and brown sugar to create the oat crumble topping.

7. Sprinkle the oat crumble topping over the date filling, covering it evenly.

8. Bake in the preheated oven for approximately 25-30 minutes or until the edges are golden brown.

9. Allow the oat and date bars to cool in the pan for at least 15-20 minutes before transferring them to a wire rack to cool completely.

10. Once cooled, cut the bars into squares or rectangles.

11. Store the oat and date bars in an airtight container at room temperature.

Chocolate Berry Smoothie Bowl

Ingredients:

For the Smoothie Base:

- 1 frozen banana
- 1 cup mixed berries (strawberries, blueberries, raspberries)

- 1/2 cup Greek yogurt

- 1 tablespoon cocoa powder

- 1 tablespoon almond butter

- 1/2 cup almond milk (or any milk of your choice)

- 1-2 teaspoons honey or maple syrup (optional, for added sweetness)

- Ice cubes (optional, for a thicker consistency)

Toppings:

- Sliced strawberries

- Fresh blueberries

- Granola

- Chia seeds

- Shredded coconut

- Dark chocolate chips or cocoa nibs

Instructions:

1. In a blender, combine the frozen banana, mixed berries, Greek yogurt, cocoa powder, almond butter, almond milk, and honey or maple syrup.

2. Blend the ingredients until smooth and creamy. If needed, add ice cubes to achieve the desired thickness.

3. Taste the smoothie base and adjust sweetness or thickness to your liking by adding more honey, maple syrup, or ice cubes.

4. Pour the chocolate berry smoothie into a bowl.

5. Arrange sliced strawberries, fresh blueberries, granola, chia seeds, shredded coconut, and dark chocolate chips or cocoa nibs on top of the smoothie base.

6. Get creative and design your smoothie bowl with a visually appealing arrangement of toppings.

7. Serve the chocolate berry smoothie bowl immediately and enjoy with a spoon.

Lemon Turmeric Coconut Bliss Balls

Ingredients:

- 1 cup shredded coconut (plus extra for rolling)
- 1/2 cup almond meal
- 1/4 cup raw cashews
- Zest of 1 lemon
- Juice of 1 lemon
- 2 tablespoons coconut oil, melted
- 2 tablespoons honey or maple syrup
- 1 teaspoon ground turmeric

- 1/2 teaspoon vanilla extract
- Pinch of salt

Instructions:

1. In a food processor, combine shredded coconut, almond meal, raw cashews, lemon zest, lemon juice, melted coconut oil, honey or maple syrup, ground turmeric, vanilla extract, and a pinch of salt.

2. Process the mixture until it forms a sticky and uniform dough.

3. Taste the mixture and adjust sweetness or tartness by adding more honey or lemon juice if desired.

4. Scoop out portions of the mixture and roll them into bite-sized bliss balls using your hands.

5. Roll each bliss ball in shredded coconut to coat the exterior.

6. Place the lemon turmeric coconut bliss balls on a tray lined with parchment paper.

7. Chill the bliss balls in the refrigerator for at least 30 minutes to firm up.

8. Once chilled, transfer the bliss balls to an airtight container and store them in the refrigerator.

9. Serve these refreshing and vibrant bliss balls as a healthy snack or dessert.

CHAPTER 9: SOUPS AND STEWS

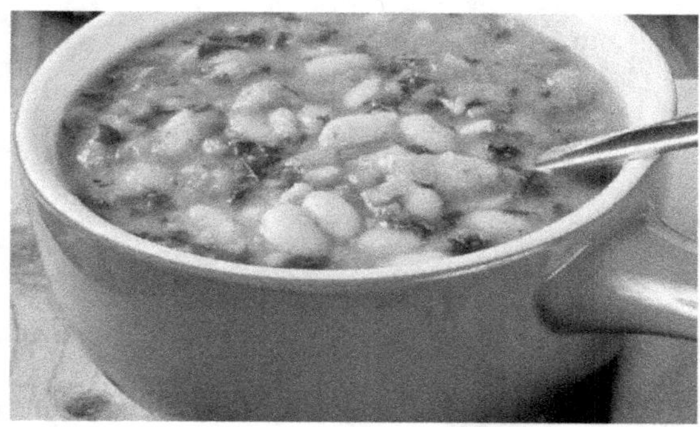

SOUPS

Turmeric Lentil Soup

Ingredients:

- 1 cup dried red lentils, rinsed and drained
- 1 onion, finely chopped
- 2 carrots, diced
- 2 celery stalks, diced
- 3 cloves garlic, minced
- 1 teaspoon ground turmeric
- 1 teaspoon ground cumin
- 1/2 teaspoon ground coriander
- 1/2 teaspoon smoked paprika
- 1/4 teaspoon cayenne pepper (optional, for heat)

- 6 cups vegetable broth
- 1 can (14 ounces) diced tomatoes
- 1 cup chopped kale or spinach
- 1 tablespoon olive oil
- Salt and black pepper to taste
- Lemon wedges for serving
- Fresh cilantro for garnish (optional)

Instructions:

1. In a large pot, heat olive oil over medium heat. Add chopped onions, carrots, and celery. Sauté for 5-7 minutes or until the vegetables are softened.

2. Add minced garlic, ground turmeric, ground cumin, ground coriander, smoked paprika, and cayenne pepper (if using). Stir well and cook for an additional 2 minutes to allow the spices to release their flavors.

3. Add rinsed red lentils to the pot and stir to coat them with the spices and vegetables.

4. Pour in vegetable broth and add diced tomatoes with their juice. Bring the soup to a boil, then reduce the heat to low, cover the pot, and let it simmer for about 20-25 minutes or until the lentils are tender.

5. Add chopped kale or spinach to the soup and simmer for an additional 5 minutes or until the greens are wilted.

6. Season the turmeric lentil soup with salt and black pepper to taste. Adjust the seasoning according to your preference.

7. Serve the soup hot, garnished with fresh cilantro if desired, and with lemon wedges on the side.

8. Enjoy this hearty and flavorful turmeric lentil soup as a nutritious and comforting meal.

Vegetable and Quinoa Minestrone

Ingredients:
- 1 cup quinoa, rinsed
- 2 tablespoons olive oil
- 1 onion, finely chopped
- 2 carrots, diced
- 2 celery stalks, diced
- 3 cloves garlic, minced
- 1 zucchini, diced
- 1 yellow squash, diced
- 1 can (14 ounces) diced tomatoes
- 1 can (15 ounces) cannellini beans, drained and rinsed

- 8 cups vegetable broth
- 1 teaspoon dried oregano
- 1 teaspoon dried basil
- 1/2 teaspoon dried thyme
- 1 bay leaf
- Salt and black pepper to taste
- 2 cups chopped kale or spinach
- 1/4 cup chopped fresh parsley
- Grated Parmesan cheese for serving (optional)

Instructions:

1. In a medium saucepan, cook the quinoa according to package instructions. Once cooked, set aside.
2. In a large pot, heat olive oil over medium heat. Add chopped onions, carrots, and celery. Sauté for 5-7 minutes or until the vegetables are softened.
3. Add minced garlic, diced zucchini, and diced yellow squash to the pot. Stir well and cook for an additional 3-4 minutes.
4. Pour in diced tomatoes with their juice and add drained cannellini beans. Stir to combine.

5. Add vegetable broth, dried oregano, dried basil, dried thyme, bay leaf, salt, and black pepper to the pot. Bring the soup to a boil, then reduce the heat to low, cover the pot, and let it simmer for about 15-20 minutes.

6. Stir in chopped kale or spinach and cook for an additional 5 minutes or until the greens are wilted.

7. Add cooked quinoa to the soup and stir to combine.

8. Taste the vegetable and quinoa minestrone and adjust the seasoning if needed.

9. Remove the bay leaf from the pot before serving.

10. Ladle the minestrone into bowls, garnish with chopped fresh parsley, and optionally sprinkle with grated Parmesan cheese.

11. Serve this hearty and nutritious vegetable and quinoa minestrone with crusty bread for a satisfying meal.

Ginger Carrot Soup

Ingredients:

- 1 tablespoon olive oil

- 1 onion, chopped
- 2 cloves garlic, minced
- 1 tablespoon fresh ginger, grated
- 1 pound (about 4 cups) carrots, peeled and sliced
- 1 medium potato, peeled and diced
- 4 cups vegetable broth
- 1 teaspoon ground turmeric
- 1/2 teaspoon ground cumin
- 1/2 teaspoon ground coriander
- 1/4 teaspoon cayenne pepper (optional, for heat)
- Salt and black pepper to taste
- 1 can (14 ounces) coconut milk
- Juice of 1 lime
- Fresh cilantro for garnish

Instructions:

1. In a large pot, heat olive oil over medium heat. Add chopped onions and sauté for 3-5 minutes until they become translucent.
2. Add minced garlic and grated ginger to the pot. Sauté for an additional 2 minutes until fragrant.
3. Add sliced carrots and diced potatoes to the pot. Stir well to coat the vegetables with the aromatics.

4. Pour in vegetable broth and bring the mixture to a boil. Reduce the heat to low, cover the pot, and let it simmer for about 15-20 minutes or until the carrots and potatoes are tender.

5. Add ground turmeric, ground cumin, ground coriander, cayenne pepper (if using), salt, and black pepper to the pot. Stir to combine.

6. Using an immersion blender, blend the soup until smooth. Alternatively, transfer the soup in batches to a blender and blend until smooth, then return it to the pot.

7. Stir in coconut milk and lime juice. Adjust the seasoning according to your taste preferences.

8. Simmer the ginger carrot soup for an additional 5 minutes to allow the flavors to meld.

9. Ladle the soup into bowls, garnish with fresh cilantro, and serve hot.

10. Enjoy this comforting and flavorful ginger carrot soup as a light and nutritious meal.

Tomato Basil Chickpea Soup

Ingredients:

- 2 tablespoons olive oil
- 1 onion, chopped

- 2 cloves garlic, minced
- 1 carrot, diced
- 1 celery stalk, diced
- 1 can (14 ounces) chickpeas, drained and rinsed
- 1 can (28 ounces) diced tomatoes
- 4 cups vegetable broth
- 1 teaspoon dried basil
- 1/2 teaspoon dried oregano
- 1/2 teaspoon dried thyme
- 1/4 teaspoon red pepper flakes (optional, for heat)
- Salt and black pepper to taste
- 1/2 cup small pasta (such as ditalini or small shells)
- 1 cup fresh spinach, chopped
- Fresh basil leaves for garnish
- Grated Parmesan cheese for serving (optional)

Instructions:

1. In a large pot, heat olive oil over medium heat. Add chopped onions and sauté for 3-5 minutes until they become translucent.

2. Add minced garlic, diced carrots, and diced celery to the pot. Sauté for an additional 5 minutes until the vegetables are slightly softened.

3. Pour in diced tomatoes with their juice, chickpeas, and vegetable broth. Bring the mixture to a boil.

4. Add dried basil, dried oregano, dried thyme, red pepper flakes (if using), salt, and black pepper to the pot. Stir to combine.

5. Reduce the heat to low, cover the pot, and let the soup simmer for about 15-20 minutes to allow the flavors to meld.

6. Add small pasta to the soup and cook according to the package instructions until al dente.

7. Stir in chopped fresh spinach and cook for an additional 2-3 minutes until the spinach wilts.

8. Taste the soup and adjust the seasoning if needed.

9. Ladle the tomato basil chickpea soup into bowls, garnish with fresh basil leaves, and optionally sprinkle with grated Parmesan cheese.

10. Serve this hearty and flavorful soup with crusty bread for a satisfying meal.

Kale and White Bean Soup

Ingredients:

- 2 tablespoons olive oil
- 1 onion, chopped
- 2 carrots, diced
- 2 celery stalks, diced
- 3 cloves garlic, minced
- 1 teaspoon dried thyme
- 1 teaspoon dried rosemary
- 1 bay leaf
- 1 can (15 ounces) white beans (cannellini or navy), drained and rinsed
- 1 bunch kale, stems removed and leaves chopped
- 4 cups vegetable broth
- 1 can (14 ounces) diced tomatoes
- Salt and black pepper to taste
- 1/2 cup small pasta (such as ditalini or small shells)
- Fresh lemon juice (optional, for serving)
- Grated Parmesan cheese for serving (optional)

Instructions:

1. In a large pot, heat olive oil over medium heat. Add chopped onions, diced carrots, and diced celery. Sauté for 5-7 minutes until the vegetables are softened.

2. Add minced garlic, dried thyme, dried rosemary, and bay leaf to the pot. Stir well and cook for an additional 2 minutes until fragrant.

3. Pour in vegetable broth, diced tomatoes with their juice, and drained white beans. Bring the mixture to a boil.

4. Reduce the heat to low, cover the pot, and let the soup simmer for about 15-20 minutes to allow the flavors to meld.

5. Add chopped kale to the soup and stir well. Simmer for an additional 5-7 minutes until the kale is tender.

6. In the last 10 minutes of cooking, add small pasta to the soup and cook according to the package instructions until al dente.

7. Remove the bay leaf from the pot and season the kale and white bean soup with salt and black pepper to taste.

8. Ladle the soup into bowls, and optionally squeeze fresh lemon juice over each serving for a burst of freshness.

9. Optionally, sprinkle grated Parmesan cheese on top of the soup before serving.

10. Enjoy this wholesome and hearty kale and white bean soup as a comforting meal.

Mushroom Barley Soup

Ingredients:

- 2 tablespoons olive oil
- 1 onion, finely chopped
- 2 carrots, diced
- 2 celery stalks, diced
- 3 cloves garlic, minced
- 8 ounces mushrooms, sliced (any variety you prefer)
- 1 cup pearl barley, rinsed
- 8 cups vegetable or mushroom broth
- 1 teaspoon dried thyme
- 1 bay leaf
- Salt and black pepper to taste
- 1/4 cup fresh parsley, chopped (for garnish)
- Lemon wedges (optional, for serving)

Instructions:

1. In a large pot, heat olive oil over medium heat. Add chopped onions, diced carrots, and diced celery. Sauté for 5-7 minutes until the vegetables are softened.

2. Add minced garlic and sliced mushrooms to the pot. Stir well and cook for an additional 5 minutes until the mushrooms release their moisture and start to brown.

3. Add rinsed pearl barley to the pot and stir to coat it with the vegetables and mushrooms.

4. Pour in vegetable or mushroom broth, add dried thyme, and toss in the bay leaf. Bring the soup to a boil.

5. Reduce the heat to low, cover the pot, and let the mushroom barley soup simmer for about 30-40 minutes or until the barley is tender.

6. Season the soup with salt and black pepper to taste. Adjust the seasoning if needed.

7. Remove the bay leaf from the pot before serving.

8. Ladle the mushroom barley soup into bowls, garnish with chopped fresh parsley, and optionally serve with lemon wedges on the side.

9. Enjoy this hearty and flavorful mushroom barley soup as a wholesome and comforting meal.

Spinach and Lentil Detox Soup

Ingredients:

- 1 cup dry green or brown lentils, rinsed and drained
- 1 tablespoon olive oil
- 1 onion, finely chopped
- 2 carrots, diced
- 3 celery stalks, diced
- 3 cloves garlic, minced
- 1 teaspoon ground cumin
- 1 teaspoon ground coriander
- 1/2 teaspoon ground turmeric
- 1/4 teaspoon cayenne pepper (optional, for heat)
- 8 cups vegetable broth
- 1 can (14 ounces) diced tomatoes
- 1 cup quinoa, rinsed
- 4 cups fresh spinach, chopped
- Juice of 1 lemon
- Salt and black pepper to taste
- Fresh cilantro or parsley for garnish (optional)

Instructions:

1. In a large pot, heat olive oil over medium heat. Add chopped onions, diced carrots, and diced celery. Sauté for 5-7 minutes until the vegetables are softened.

2. Add minced garlic, ground cumin, ground coriander, ground turmeric, and cayenne pepper (if using). Stir well and cook for an additional 2 minutes until the spices are fragrant.

3. Add rinsed lentils to the pot and stir to combine with the vegetables and spices.

4. Pour in vegetable broth, diced tomatoes with their juice, and rinsed quinoa. Bring the mixture to a boil.

5. Reduce the heat to low, cover the pot, and let the soup simmer for about 25-30 minutes or until the lentils and quinoa are tender.

6. Stir in chopped fresh spinach and cook for an additional 3-5 minutes until the spinach wilts.

7. Squeeze the juice of one lemon into the soup and stir to incorporate.

8. Season the spinach and lentil detox soup with salt and black pepper to taste. Adjust the seasoning if needed.

9. Ladle the soup into bowls, garnish with fresh cilantro or parsley if desired, and serve hot.

10. Enjoy this nutrient-rich and detoxifying spinach and lentil soup as a nourishing and flavorful meal.

Butternut Squash and Apple Soup

Ingredients:

- 1 medium-sized butternut squash, peeled, seeded, and diced
- 2 apples, peeled, cored, and chopped
- 1 onion, chopped
- 2 carrots, peeled and chopped
- 3 cups vegetable broth
- 1 cup apple juice or apple cider
- 1 teaspoon ground cinnamon
- 1/2 teaspoon ground nutmeg
- 1/4 teaspoon ground ginger
- 1/4 teaspoon ground cloves
- Salt and black pepper to taste
- 2 tablespoons olive oil
- Optional toppings: roasted pumpkin seeds, a drizzle of cream, or a sprinkle of chopped fresh parsley

Instructions:

1. Preheat your oven to 400°F (200°C).

2. Place the diced butternut squash, chopped apples, chopped onion, and chopped carrots on a baking sheet. Drizzle with olive oil and toss to coat the vegetables and apples evenly.

3. Roast the vegetables and apples in the preheated oven for about 30-35 minutes or until they are tender and slightly caramelized.

4. In a large pot, combine the roasted butternut squash, apples, onion, and carrots. Add vegetable broth, apple juice or cider, ground cinnamon, ground nutmeg, ground ginger, and ground cloves.

5. Bring the mixture to a boil, then reduce the heat to low, cover the pot, and let it simmer for about 15-20 minutes to allow the flavors to meld.

6. Use an immersion blender to puree the soup until smooth. Alternatively, transfer the soup to a blender in batches, blending until smooth, then return it to the pot.

7. Season the butternut squash and apple soup with salt and black pepper to taste. Adjust the seasoning if needed.

8. If the soup is too thick, you can add more vegetable broth or apple juice to reach your desired consistency.

9. Serve the soup hot, garnished with your choice of toppings, such as roasted pumpkin seeds, a drizzle of cream, or chopped fresh parsley.

10. Enjoy this comforting and flavorful butternut squash and apple soup as a delightful fall or winter meal.

Turmeric Cauliflower Soup

Ingredients:

- 1 large cauliflower, cut into florets
- 1 onion, chopped
- 3 cloves garlic, minced
- 1 tablespoon fresh turmeric, grated (or 1 teaspoon ground turmeric)
- 1 teaspoon ground cumin
- 1/2 teaspoon ground coriander
- 1/4 teaspoon cayenne pepper (optional, for heat)
- 4 cups vegetable broth
- 1 can (14 ounces) coconut milk
- 2 tablespoons olive oil
- Salt and black pepper to taste

- Fresh cilantro for garnish

- Lime wedges for serving

Instructions:

1. Preheat your oven to 400°F (200°C).

2. Place cauliflower florets on a baking sheet, drizzle with olive oil, and season with salt and black pepper. Roast in the preheated oven for about 25-30 minutes or until the cauliflower is tender and golden brown.

3. In a large pot, heat olive oil over medium heat. Add chopped onions and sauté for 5-7 minutes until they become translucent.

4. Add minced garlic, grated fresh turmeric (or ground turmeric), ground cumin, ground coriander, and cayenne pepper (if using). Stir well and cook for an additional 2 minutes until the spices are fragrant.

5. Add roasted cauliflower to the pot and pour in vegetable broth. Bring the mixture to a boil, then reduce the heat to low, cover the pot, and let it simmer for about 15-20 minutes.

6. Use an immersion blender to puree the soup until smooth. Alternatively, transfer the soup to a blender in batches, blending until smooth, then return it to the pot.

7. Stir in coconut milk and simmer for an additional 5-7 minutes to allow the flavors to meld.

8. Season the turmeric cauliflower soup with salt and black pepper to taste. Adjust the seasoning if needed.

9. Ladle the soup into bowls, garnish with fresh cilantro, and serve with lime wedges on the side.

10. Enjoy this vibrant and nutritious turmeric cauliflower soup as a comforting and flavorful meal.

Cabbage and Turmeric Chicken Soup

Ingredients:

- 1 pound boneless, skinless chicken breasts, diced
- 1 tablespoon olive oil
- 1 onion, chopped
- 3 cloves garlic, minced

- 1 tablespoon fresh turmeric, grated (or 1 teaspoon ground turmeric)
- 1 teaspoon ground cumin
- 1/2 teaspoon ground coriander
- 1/4 teaspoon cayenne pepper (optional, for heat)
- 4 cups cabbage, thinly sliced
- 2 carrots, sliced
- 8 cups chicken broth
- 1 cup quinoa, rinsed
- Salt and black pepper to taste
- Fresh cilantro for garnish
- Lemon wedges for serving

Instructions:

1. In a large pot, heat olive oil over medium heat. Add diced chicken and cook until browned on all sides. Remove the chicken from the pot and set it aside.
2. In the same pot, add chopped onions and sauté for 5-7 minutes until they become translucent.
3. Add minced garlic, grated fresh turmeric (or ground turmeric), ground cumin, ground coriander, and cayenne pepper (if using). Stir well and cook for an additional 2 minutes until the spices are fragrant.

4. Add sliced cabbage and carrots to the pot. Stir and cook for about 5 minutes until the vegetables begin to soften.

5. Pour in chicken broth and bring the mixture to a boil. Reduce the heat to low, cover the pot, and let it simmer for about 15-20 minutes.

6. Stir in quinoa and the cooked diced chicken. Simmer for an additional 15-20 minutes or until the quinoa is cooked through.

7. Season the cabbage and turmeric chicken soup with salt and black pepper to taste. Adjust the seasoning if needed.

8. Ladle the soup into bowls, garnish with fresh cilantro, and serve with lemon wedges on the side.

9. Enjoy this hearty and flavorful cabbage and turmeric chicken soup as a comforting and nutritious meal.

Lemon Garlic Chickpea Soup

Ingredients:

- 2 tablespoons olive oil
- 1 onion, finely chopped
- 3 cloves garlic, minced

- 2 carrots, diced
- 2 celery stalks, diced
- 2 cans (15 ounces each) chickpeas, drained and rinsed
- 6 cups vegetable broth
- 1 lemon, zest and juice
- 1 teaspoon dried thyme
- 1/2 teaspoon dried rosemary
- Salt and black pepper to taste
- 1/2 cup small pasta (such as ditalini or small shells)
- Fresh parsley for garnish
- Grated Parmesan cheese for serving (optional)

Instructions:

1. In a large pot, heat olive oil over medium heat. Add chopped onions, diced carrots, and diced celery. Sauté for 5-7 minutes until the vegetables are softened.

2. Add minced garlic to the pot and stir well. Cook for an additional 2 minutes until the garlic is fragrant.

3. Pour in vegetable broth, add drained chickpeas, dried thyme, dried rosemary, and the zest and juice of one lemon. Bring the mixture to a boil.

4. Reduce the heat to low, cover the pot, and let the soup simmer for about 15-20 minutes to allow the flavors to meld.

5. In the last 10 minutes of cooking, add small pasta to the soup and cook according to the package instructions until al dente.

6. Season the lemon garlic chickpea soup with salt and black pepper to taste. Adjust the seasoning if needed.

7. Ladle the soup into bowls, garnish with fresh parsley, and optionally serve with grated Parmesan cheese on the side.

8. Enjoy this refreshing and flavorful lemon garlic chickpea soup as a light and satisfying meal.

Sweet Potato and Ginger Soup

Ingredients:

- 2 tablespoons olive oil
- 1 onion, chopped
- 3 cloves garlic, minced
- 1 tablespoon fresh ginger, grated
- 3 large sweet potatoes, peeled and diced
- 4 cups vegetable broth
- 1 can (14 ounces) coconut milk

- 1 teaspoon ground cumin

- 1/2 teaspoon ground coriander

- 1/4 teaspoon cayenne pepper (optional, for heat)

- Salt and black pepper to taste

- Fresh cilantro for garnish

- Roasted pumpkin seeds for topping (optional)

Instructions:

1. In a large pot, heat olive oil over medium heat. Add chopped onions and sauté for 5-7 minutes until they become translucent.

2. Add minced garlic and grated fresh ginger to the pot. Stir well and cook for an additional 2 minutes until the ginger is fragrant.

3. Add diced sweet potatoes to the pot and pour in vegetable broth. Bring the mixture to a boil.

4. Reduce the heat to low, cover the pot, and let the sweet potato and ginger soup simmer for about 20-25 minutes or until the sweet potatoes are tender.

5. Use an immersion blender to puree the soup until smooth. Alternatively, transfer the soup to a blender in batches, blending until smooth, then return it to the pot.

6. Stir in coconut milk, ground cumin, ground coriander, and cayenne pepper (if using). Simmer for an additional 5-7 minutes to allow the flavors to meld.

7. Season the sweet potato and ginger soup with salt and black pepper to taste. Adjust the seasoning if needed.

8. Ladle the soup into bowls, garnish with fresh cilantro, and optionally top with roasted pumpkin seeds.

9. Enjoy this velvety and aromatic sweet potato and ginger soup as a comforting and nourishing meal.

STEWS

Turmeric Chicken and Vegetable Stew

Ingredients:

- 1.5 pounds boneless, skinless chicken thighs, cut into bite-sized pieces
- 2 tablespoons olive oil
- 1 onion, chopped
- 3 cloves garlic, minced

- 1 tablespoon fresh turmeric, grated (or 1 teaspoon ground turmeric)
- 1 teaspoon ground cumin
- 1 teaspoon ground coriander
- 1/2 teaspoon cayenne pepper (optional, for heat)
- 3 carrots, peeled and sliced
- 3 celery stalks, sliced
- 1 sweet potato, peeled and diced
- 1 bell pepper, diced
- 4 cups chicken broth
- 1 can (14 ounces) diced tomatoes
- 1 cup green beans, trimmed and chopped
- Salt and black pepper to taste
- 1/4 cup chopped fresh cilantro for garnish

Instructions:

1. In a large pot, heat olive oil over medium heat. Add chopped onions and sauté for 5-7 minutes until they become translucent.

2. Add minced garlic, grated fresh turmeric (or ground turmeric), ground cumin, ground coriander, and cayenne pepper (if using). Stir well and cook for an additional 2 minutes until the spices are fragrant.

3. Add chicken pieces to the pot and brown them on all sides. This should take about 5-7 minutes.

4. Once the chicken is browned, add sliced carrots, sliced celery, diced sweet potato, and diced bell pepper to the pot. Stir to combine.

5. Pour in chicken broth and diced tomatoes with their juice. Bring the mixture to a boil.

6. Reduce the heat to low, cover the pot, and let the stew simmer for about 20-25 minutes or until the vegetables are tender and the chicken is cooked through.

7. Add chopped green beans to the stew and simmer for an additional 5-7 minutes until the beans are cooked but still slightly crisp.

8. Season the turmeric chicken and vegetable stew with salt and black pepper to taste. Adjust the seasoning if needed.

9. Ladle the stew into bowls, garnish with chopped fresh cilantro, and serve hot.

10. Enjoy this hearty and flavorful turmeric chicken and vegetable stew as a comforting and nutritious meal.

Quinoa and Kale Lentil Stew

Ingredients:

- 1 cup quinoa, rinsed
- 1 cup green or brown lentils, rinsed and drained
- 2 tablespoons olive oil
- 1 onion, chopped
- 3 cloves garlic, minced
- 1 teaspoon ground cumin
- 1 teaspoon ground coriander
- 1/2 teaspoon smoked paprika
- 1/4 teaspoon cayenne pepper (optional, for heat)
- 1 can (14 ounces) diced tomatoes
- 6 cups vegetable broth
- 4 cups chopped kale, stems removed
- Salt and black pepper to taste
- Juice of 1 lemon
- Fresh parsley for garnish

Instructions:

1. In a medium saucepan, combine rinsed quinoa with 2 cups of water. Bring to a boil, then reduce the heat to low, cover, and let it simmer for about 15 minutes or until the quinoa is cooked and water is absorbed. Set aside.

2. In a large pot, heat olive oil over medium heat. Add chopped onions and sauté for 5-7 minutes until they become translucent.

3. Add minced garlic, ground cumin, ground coriander, smoked paprika, and cayenne pepper (if using). Stir well and cook for an additional 2 minutes until the spices are fragrant.

4. Add rinsed lentils, diced tomatoes with their juice, and vegetable broth to the pot. Bring the mixture to a boil.

5. Reduce the heat to low, cover the pot, and let the lentil stew simmer for about 25-30 minutes or until the lentils are tender.

6. Stir in chopped kale and cook for an additional 5-7 minutes until the kale is wilted.

7. Season the quinoa and kale lentil stew with salt and black pepper to taste. Adjust the seasoning if needed.

8. Stir in the cooked quinoa and squeeze the juice of one lemon into the stew. Mix well.

9. Ladle the stew into bowls, garnish with fresh parsley, and serve hot.

10. Enjoy this nutritious and hearty quinoa and kale lentil stew as a flavorful and satisfying meal.

Ginger-Turmeric Beef Stew

Ingredients:

- 1.5 pounds beef stew meat, cut into bite-sized pieces
- 2 tablespoons olive oil
- 1 onion, chopped
- 3 cloves garlic, minced
- 1 tablespoon fresh ginger, grated
- 1 tablespoon fresh turmeric, grated (or 1 teaspoon ground turmeric)
- 1 teaspoon ground cumin
- 1 teaspoon ground coriander
- 1/4 teaspoon cayenne pepper (optional, for heat)
- 4 cups beef broth
- 2 carrots, peeled and sliced
- 2 parsnips, peeled and sliced
- 2 potatoes, peeled and diced
- 1 cup green beans, trimmed and chopped
- Salt and black pepper to taste
- Fresh cilantro for garnish
- Cooked rice or crusty bread for serving

Instructions:

1. In a large pot, heat olive oil over medium heat. Add beef stew meat and brown it on all sides. This should take about 5-7 minutes.

2. Once the beef is browned, add chopped onions and sauté for 5-7 minutes until they become translucent.

3. Add minced garlic, grated fresh ginger, grated fresh turmeric (or ground turmeric), ground cumin, ground coriander, and cayenne pepper (if using). Stir well and cook for an additional 2 minutes until the spices are fragrant.

4. Pour in beef broth and bring the mixture to a boil.

5. Reduce the heat to low, cover the pot, and let the beef stew simmer for about 1.5 to 2 hours or until the beef is tender.

6. Add sliced carrots, sliced parsnips, diced potatoes, and chopped green beans to the stew. Continue to simmer for an additional 20-25 minutes or until the vegetables are cooked through.

7. Season the ginger-turmeric beef stew with salt and black pepper to taste. Adjust the seasoning if needed.

8. Ladle the stew into bowls, garnish with fresh cilantro, and serve hot over cooked rice or with crusty bread on the side.

9. Enjoy this warming and flavorful ginger-turmeric beef stew as a hearty and satisfying meal.

Chickpea and Spinach Stew

Ingredients:

- 2 tablespoons olive oil
- 1 onion, chopped
- 3 cloves garlic, minced
- 1 teaspoon ground cumin
- 1 teaspoon ground coriander
- 1/2 teaspoon smoked paprika
- 1/4 teaspoon cayenne pepper (optional, for heat)
- 2 cans (15 ounces each) chickpeas, drained and rinsed
- 1 can (14 ounces) diced tomatoes
- 4 cups vegetable broth
- 1 teaspoon lemon zest

- Juice of 1 lemon
- 6 cups fresh spinach, chopped
- Salt and black pepper to taste
- Fresh parsley for garnish
- Cooked couscous or rice for serving

Instructions:

1. In a large pot, heat olive oil over medium heat. Add chopped onions and sauté for 5-7 minutes until they become translucent.

2. Add minced garlic, ground cumin, ground coriander, smoked paprika, and cayenne pepper (if using). Stir well and cook for an additional 2 minutes until the spices are fragrant.

3. Add drained chickpeas, diced tomatoes with their juice, and vegetable broth to the pot. Bring the mixture to a boil.

4. Reduce the heat to low, cover the pot, and let the chickpea and spinach stew simmer for about 15-20 minutes.

5. Stir in lemon zest, lemon juice, and chopped fresh spinach. Cook for an additional 5-7 minutes until the spinach is wilted.

6. Season the stew with salt and black pepper to taste. Adjust the seasoning if needed.

7. Ladle the stew into bowls, garnish with fresh parsley, and serve hot over cooked couscous or rice.

8. Enjoy this wholesome and flavorful chickpea and spinach stew as a nourishing and satisfying meal.

Butternut Squash and Lentil Stew

Ingredients:

- 2 tablespoons olive oil
- 1 onion, chopped
- 3 cloves garlic, minced
- 1 butternut squash, peeled, seeded, and diced
- 1 cup dry green or brown lentils, rinsed and drained
- 1 teaspoon ground cumin
- 1 teaspoon ground coriander
- 1/2 teaspoon smoked paprika
- 1/4 teaspoon cayenne pepper (optional, for heat)
- 4 cups vegetable broth
- 1 can (14 ounces) diced tomatoes
- Salt and black pepper to taste
- Fresh parsley for garnish

- Greek yogurt or coconut cream for serving (optional)

Instructions:

1. In a large pot, heat olive oil over medium heat. Add chopped onions and sauté for 5-7 minutes until they become translucent.

2. Add minced garlic, diced butternut squash, rinsed lentils, ground cumin, ground coriander, smoked paprika, and cayenne pepper (if using). Stir well and cook for an additional 5 minutes until the spices are fragrant.

3. Pour in vegetable broth and diced tomatoes with their juice. Bring the mixture to a boil.

4. Reduce the heat to low, cover the pot, and let the butternut squash and lentil stew simmer for about 25-30 minutes or until the lentils are tender and the squash is cooked through.

5. Season the stew with salt and black pepper to taste. Adjust the seasoning if needed.

6. Ladle the stew into bowls, garnish with fresh parsley, and optionally serve with a dollop of Greek yogurt or a drizzle of coconut cream.

7. Enjoy this hearty and flavorful butternut squash and lentil stew as a comforting and nutritious meal.

Cauliflower and Chickpea Curry Stew

Ingredients:

- 2 tablespoons coconut oil
- 1 onion, chopped
- 3 cloves garlic, minced
- 1 tablespoon fresh ginger, grated
- 1 tablespoon curry powder
- 1 teaspoon ground cumin
- 1 teaspoon ground coriander
- 1/2 teaspoon turmeric powder
- 1/4 teaspoon cayenne pepper (optional, for heat)
- 1 can (15 ounces) chickpeas, drained and rinsed
- 1 cauliflower, cut into florets
- 1 can (14 ounces) diced tomatoes
- 1 can (14 ounces) coconut milk
- 1 cup vegetable broth
- Salt and black pepper to taste
- Fresh cilantro for garnish
- Cooked basmati rice for serving

Instructions:

1. In a large pot, heat coconut oil over medium heat. Add chopped onions and sauté for 5-7 minutes until they become translucent.

2. Add minced garlic and grated fresh ginger to the pot. Stir well and cook for an additional 2 minutes until the ginger is fragrant.

3. Add curry powder, ground cumin, ground coriander, turmeric powder, and cayenne pepper (if using). Stir the spices into the onions, garlic, and ginger.

4. Add drained chickpeas, cauliflower florets, diced tomatoes with their juice, coconut milk, and vegetable broth to the pot. Bring the mixture to a boil.

5. Reduce the heat to low, cover the pot, and let the cauliflower and chickpea curry stew simmer for about 20-25 minutes or until the cauliflower is tender.

6. Season the stew with salt and black pepper to taste. Adjust the seasoning if needed.

7. Serve the cauliflower and chickpea curry stew over cooked basmati rice.

8. Garnish with fresh cilantro before serving.

9. Enjoy this flavorful and aromatic cauliflower and chickpea curry stew as a delicious and satisfying meal.

Mushroom Barley Vegetable Stew

Ingredients:

- 2 tablespoons olive oil
- 1 onion, chopped
- 3 cloves garlic, minced
- 8 ounces cremini mushrooms, sliced
- 8 ounces shiitake mushrooms, stemmed and sliced
- 1 cup pearl barley, rinsed
- 4 carrots, peeled and diced
- 3 celery stalks, diced
- 1 parsnip, peeled and diced
- 1 can (14 ounces) diced tomatoes
- 8 cups vegetable broth
- 2 bay leaves
- 1 teaspoon dried thyme
- Salt and black pepper to taste
- Fresh parsley for garnish

Instructions:

1. In a large pot, heat olive oil over medium heat. Add chopped onions and sauté for 5-7 minutes until they become translucent.

2. Add minced garlic, sliced cremini mushrooms, and sliced shiitake mushrooms. Stir well and cook for an additional 5 minutes until the mushrooms are softened.

3. Add rinsed pearl barley to the pot and stir to coat it with the mushrooms and onions.

4. Pour in vegetable broth, diced tomatoes with their juice, diced carrots, diced celery, diced parsnip, bay leaves, and dried thyme. Bring the mixture to a boil.

5. Reduce the heat to low, cover the pot, and let the mushroom barley vegetable stew simmer for about 30-35 minutes or until the barley is tender.

6. Season the stew with salt and black pepper to taste. Adjust the seasoning if needed.

7. Remove the bay leaves from the stew before serving.

8. Ladle the stew into bowls, garnish with fresh parsley, and serve hot.

9. Enjoy this hearty and wholesome mushroom barley vegetable stew as a comforting and nutritious meal.

Tomato Basil Cannellini Bean Stew

Ingredients:

- 2 tablespoons olive oil
- 1 onion, chopped
- 3 cloves garlic, minced
- 1 can (15 ounces) cannellini beans, drained and rinsed
- 1 can (14 ounces) diced tomatoes
- 1 can (6 ounces) tomato paste
- 4 cups vegetable broth
- 1 teaspoon dried basil
- 1 teaspoon dried oregano
- 1/2 teaspoon dried thyme
- 1/4 teaspoon red pepper flakes (optional, for heat)
- Salt and black pepper to taste
- Fresh basil leaves for garnish
- Grated Parmesan cheese for serving (optional)

Instructions:

1. In a large pot, heat olive oil over medium heat. Add chopped onions and sauté for 5-7 minutes until they become translucent.

2. Add minced garlic to the pot and stir well. Cook for an additional 2 minutes until the garlic is fragrant.

3. Pour in vegetable broth, diced tomatoes with their juice, and tomato paste. Stir to combine.

4. Add drained cannellini beans to the pot and stir again.

5. Season the stew with dried basil, dried oregano, dried thyme, red pepper flakes (if using), salt, and black pepper. Stir well to incorporate the herbs and spices.

6. Bring the mixture to a boil, then reduce the heat to low, cover the pot, and let the tomato basil cannellini bean stew simmer for about 15-20 minutes.

7. Taste and adjust the seasoning if needed.

8. Ladle the stew into bowls, garnish with fresh basil leaves, and optionally serve with grated Parmesan cheese on the side.

9. Enjoy this flavorful and comforting tomato basil cannellini bean stew as a light and satisfying meal.

Sweet Potato and Black Bean Chili Stew

Ingredients:

- 2 tablespoons olive oil
- 1 onion, chopped
- 3 cloves garlic, minced
- 2 sweet potatoes, peeled and diced
- 1 red bell pepper, diced
- 1 green bell pepper, diced
- 1 jalapeño pepper, seeded and minced (optional, for heat)
- 2 teaspoons ground cumin
- 1 teaspoon chili powder
- 1/2 teaspoon smoked paprika
- 1/4 teaspoon cayenne pepper (optional, for extra heat)
- 2 cans (15 ounces each) black beans, drained and rinsed
- 1 can (14 ounces) diced tomatoes
- 4 cups vegetable broth

- Salt and black pepper to taste
- Juice of 1 lime
- Fresh cilantro for garnish
- Avocado slices for serving (optional)

Instructions:

1. In a large pot, heat olive oil over medium heat. Add chopped onions and sauté for 5-7 minutes until they become translucent.

2. Add minced garlic, diced sweet potatoes, diced red bell pepper, diced green bell pepper, and minced jalapeño pepper (if using). Stir well and cook for an additional 5 minutes until the vegetables begin to soften.

3. Add ground cumin, chili powder, smoked paprika, and cayenne pepper (if using). Stir the spices into the vegetables.

4. Pour in vegetable broth, diced tomatoes with their juice, and drained black beans. Bring the mixture to a boil.

5. Reduce the heat to low, cover the pot, and let the sweet potato and black bean chili stew simmer for about 20-25 minutes or until the sweet potatoes are tender.

6. Season the stew with salt and black pepper to taste. Adjust the seasoning if needed.

7. Stir in the lime juice just before serving.

8. Ladle the stew into bowls, garnish with fresh cilantro, and optionally serve with avocado slices on the side.

9. Enjoy this hearty and flavorful sweet potato and black bean chili stew as a nutritious and satisfying meal.

Chicken and Quinoa Stew with Lemon

Ingredients:

- 2 tablespoons olive oil
- 1 onion, chopped
- 3 cloves garlic, minced
- 1 pound boneless, skinless chicken thighs, cut into bite-sized pieces
- 1 cup quinoa, rinsed
- 4 cups chicken broth
- 1 lemon, zest and juice
- 2 carrots, peeled and diced
- 2 celery stalks, diced
- 1 parsnip, peeled and diced
- 1 teaspoon dried thyme

- Salt and black pepper to taste
- Fresh parsley for garnish

Instructions:

1. In a large pot, heat olive oil over medium heat. Add chopped onions and sauté for 5-7 minutes until they become translucent.
2. Add minced garlic to the pot and stir well. Cook for an additional 2 minutes until the garlic is fragrant.
3. Add chicken pieces to the pot and brown them on all sides. This should take about 5-7 minutes.
4. Once the chicken is browned, add rinsed quinoa, chicken broth, lemon zest, and lemon juice to the pot. Stir well.
5. Add diced carrots, diced celery, diced parsnip, dried thyme, salt, and black pepper to the pot. Bring the mixture to a boil.
6. Reduce the heat to low, cover the pot, and let the chicken and quinoa stew simmer for about 20-25 minutes or until the quinoa is cooked and the vegetables are tender.
7. Taste and adjust the seasoning if needed.
8. Ladle the stew into bowls, garnish with fresh parsley, and serve hot.

9. Enjoy this light and flavorful chicken and quinoa stew with lemon as a nourishing and satisfying meal.

Red Lentil and Vegetable Coconut Stew

Ingredients:

- 2 tablespoons coconut oil
- 1 onion, chopped
- 3 cloves garlic, minced
- 1 tablespoon fresh ginger, grated
- 1 tablespoon red curry paste
- 1 cup red lentils, rinsed and drained
- 1 can (14 ounces) diced tomatoes
- 1 can (14 ounces) coconut milk
- 4 cups vegetable broth
- 2 carrots, peeled and sliced
- 1 bell pepper, diced
- 1 zucchini, diced
- 1 teaspoon ground cumin
- 1 teaspoon ground coriander
- 1/2 teaspoon turmeric powder
- Salt and black pepper to taste
- Juice of 1 lime
- Fresh cilantro for garnish

- Cooked basmati rice for serving

Instructions:

1. In a large pot, heat coconut oil over medium heat. Add chopped onions and sauté for 5-7 minutes until they become translucent.
2. Add minced garlic and grated fresh ginger to the pot. Stir well and cook for an additional 2 minutes until the ginger is fragrant.
3. Add red curry paste, ground cumin, ground coriander, and turmeric powder. Stir the spices into the onions, garlic, and ginger.
4. Pour in vegetable broth, diced tomatoes with their juice, and coconut milk. Stir to combine.
5. Add rinsed red lentils, sliced carrots, diced bell pepper, and diced zucchini to the pot. Bring the mixture to a boil.
6. Reduce the heat to low, cover the pot, and let the red lentil and vegetable coconut stew simmer for about 20-25 minutes or until the lentils are tender.
7. Season the stew with salt and black pepper to taste. Adjust the seasoning if needed.
8. Stir in the lime juice just before serving.

9. Ladle the stew into bowls, garnish with fresh cilantro, and serve over cooked basmati rice.

10. Enjoy this flavorful and aromatic red lentil and vegetable coconut stew as a satisfying and wholesome meal.

Spinach and Turkey Meatball Stew

Ingredients:

For Turkey Meatballs:

- 1 pound ground turkey
- 1/2 cup breadcrumbs
- 1/4 cup grated Parmesan cheese
- 1 egg
- 2 cloves garlic, minced
- 1 teaspoon dried oregano
- 1 teaspoon dried basil
- Salt and black pepper to taste

For Stew:

- 2 tablespoons olive oil
- 1 onion, chopped
- 3 cloves garlic, minced
- 1 can (14 ounces) diced tomatoes
- 4 cups chicken broth
- 1 teaspoon dried thyme

- 1 teaspoon dried rosemary
- 1 bay leaf
- 4 cups fresh spinach, chopped
- Salt and black pepper to taste
- Fresh parsley for garnish
- Cooked quinoa or pasta for serving

Instructions:

For Turkey Meatballs:

1. Preheat the oven to 375°F (190°C).
2. In a large bowl, combine ground turkey, breadcrumbs, grated Parmesan cheese, egg, minced garlic, dried oregano, dried basil, salt, and black pepper.
3. Mix the ingredients until well combined.
4. Shape the mixture into meatballs, approximately 1 inch in diameter.
5. Place the meatballs on a baking sheet lined with parchment paper.
6. Bake in the preheated oven for 20-25 minutes or until the meatballs are cooked through and browned on the outside.

For Stew:

1. In a large pot, heat olive oil over medium heat. Add chopped onions and sauté for 5-7 minutes until they become translucent.
2. Add minced garlic to the pot and stir well. Cook for an additional 2 minutes until the garlic is fragrant.
3. Pour in chicken broth and diced tomatoes with their juice. Add dried thyme, dried rosemary, and a bay leaf. Stir to combine.
4. Gently drop the baked turkey meatballs into the stew.
5. Bring the mixture to a boil, then reduce the heat to low, cover the pot, and let the stew simmer for about 15-20 minutes.
6. Add chopped fresh spinach to the pot and cook for an additional 5-7 minutes until the spinach is wilted.
7. Season the stew with salt and black pepper to taste. Adjust the seasoning if needed.
8. Remove the bay leaf from the stew before serving.

9. Ladle the stew into bowls, garnish with fresh parsley, and serve over cooked quinoa or pasta.

10. Enjoy this wholesome and comforting spinach and turkey meatball stew as a flavorful and nutritious meal.

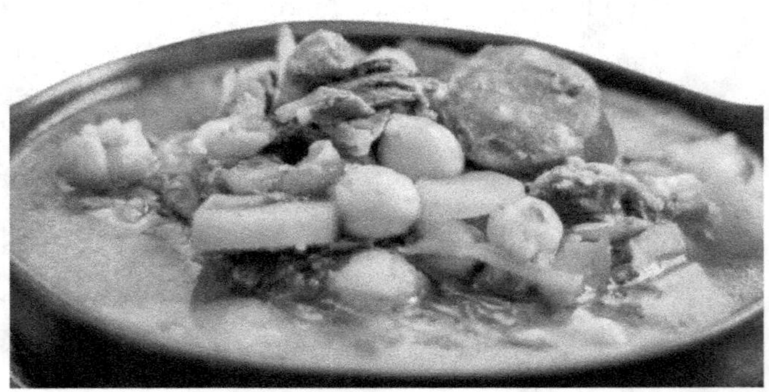

CHAPTER 10: SMOOTHIES

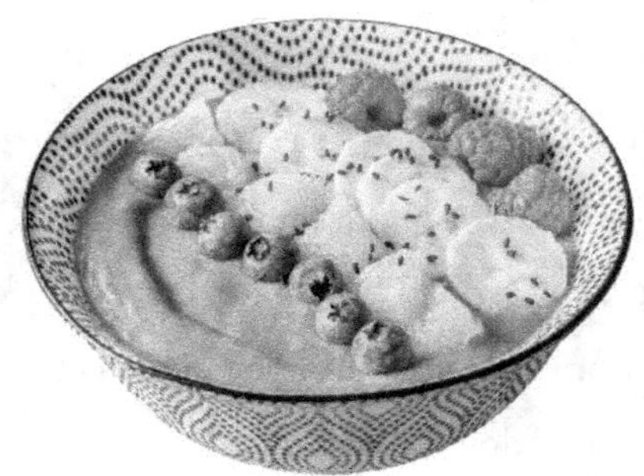

Turmeric Mango Smoothie

Ingredients:

- 1 cup frozen mango chunks
- 1 banana, peeled and sliced
- 1/2 cup Greek yogurt
- 1/2 cup coconut milk
- 1/2 teaspoon turmeric powder
- 1/2 teaspoon grated fresh ginger
- 1 tablespoon honey or maple syrup (optional, for sweetness)
- Ice cubes (optional)

Instructions:

1. Place frozen mango chunks, sliced banana, Greek yogurt, coconut milk, turmeric powder, grated fresh ginger, and honey (if using) in a blender.

2. Blend the ingredients on high speed until smooth and creamy. If the smoothie is too thick, you can add more coconut milk or a splash of water to reach your desired consistency.

3. Taste the smoothie and adjust the sweetness by adding more honey or maple syrup if needed.

4. If you prefer a colder smoothie, you can add ice cubes and blend again until well combined.

5. Pour the turmeric mango smoothie into glasses.

6. Optionally, garnish with a sprinkle of turmeric powder or a slice of fresh mango.

7. Enjoy this vibrant and refreshing turmeric mango smoothie as a nutritious and delicious drink!

Berry Spinach Avocado Smoothie

Ingredients:

- 1 cup fresh spinach leaves
- 1/2 avocado, peeled and pitted

- 1/2 cup mixed berries (such as strawberries, blueberries, raspberries)
- 1 banana, peeled
- 1/2 cup Greek yogurt
- 1 cup almond milk (or any milk of your choice)
- 1 tablespoon chia seeds (optional)
- 1 tablespoon honey or maple syrup (optional, for sweetness)
- Ice cubes (optional)

Instructions:

1. Place fresh spinach leaves, peeled and pitted avocado, mixed berries, peeled banana, Greek yogurt, almond milk, chia seeds (if using), and honey or maple syrup (if using) in a blender.
2. Blend the ingredients on high speed until smooth and creamy. If the smoothie is too thick, you can add more almond milk or a splash of water to reach your desired consistency.
3. Taste the smoothie and adjust the sweetness by adding more honey or maple syrup if needed.
4. If you prefer a colder smoothie, you can add ice cubes and blend again until well combined.
5. Pour the berry spinach avocado smoothie into glasses.

6. Optionally, garnish with a few whole berries or a slice of avocado.

7. Enjoy this nutrient-packed and delicious berry spinach avocado smoothie as a refreshing and wholesome drink!

Green Tea Citrus Smoothie

Ingredients:

- 1 cup brewed green tea, cooled
- 1/2 cup orange juice
- 1 banana, peeled
- 1 cup fresh spinach leaves
- 1/2 cup Greek yogurt
- 1 tablespoon honey or maple syrup (optional, for sweetness)
- Ice cubes (optional)

Instructions:

1. Brew green tea and allow it to cool. You can speed up the cooling process by placing it in the refrigerator for a few minutes.

2. In a blender, combine cooled green tea, orange juice, peeled banana, fresh spinach leaves, Greek yogurt, and honey or maple syrup (if using).

3. Blend the ingredients on high speed until smooth and well combined. If the smoothie is too thick, you can add more green tea or a splash of water to reach your desired consistency.
4. Taste the smoothie and adjust the sweetness by adding more honey or maple syrup if needed.
5. If you prefer a colder smoothie, you can add ice cubes and blend again until well combined.
6. Pour the green tea citrus smoothie into glasses.
7. Optionally, garnish with a slice of orange or a sprig of mint.
8. Enjoy this refreshing and antioxidant-rich green tea citrus smoothie as a revitalizing and healthy beverage!

Pineapple Ginger Turmeric Smoothie

Ingredients:

- 1 cup pineapple chunks (fresh or frozen)
- 1 banana, peeled
- 1/2 teaspoon grated fresh ginger
- 1/2 teaspoon ground turmeric
- 1 cup coconut water or water
- 1/2 cup Greek yogurt
- 1 tablespoon chia seeds (optional)

- 1 tablespoon honey or maple syrup (optional, for sweetness)
- Ice cubes (optional)

Instructions:

1. Place pineapple chunks, peeled banana, grated fresh ginger, ground turmeric, coconut water or water, Greek yogurt, chia seeds (if using), and honey or maple syrup (if using) in a blender.

2. Blend the ingredients on high speed until smooth and well combined. If the smoothie is too thick, you can add more coconut water or water to reach your desired consistency.

3. Taste the smoothie and adjust the sweetness by adding more honey or maple syrup if needed.

4. If you prefer a colder smoothie, you can add ice cubes and blend again until well combined.

5. Pour the pineapple ginger turmeric smoothie into glasses.

6. Optionally, garnish with a slice of pineapple or a sprinkle of turmeric.

7. Enjoy this tropical and anti-inflammatory pineapple ginger turmeric smoothie as a flavorful and healthful beverage!

Blueberry Almond Butter Smoothie

Ingredients:

- 1 cup blueberries (fresh or frozen)
- 1 banana, peeled
- 2 tablespoons almond butter
- 1 cup almond milk (or any milk of your choice)
- 1/2 cup Greek yogurt
- 1 tablespoon chia seeds (optional)
- 1 tablespoon honey or maple syrup (optional, for sweetness)
- Ice cubes (optional)

Instructions:

1. Place blueberries, peeled banana, almond butter, almond milk, Greek yogurt, chia seeds (if using), and honey or maple syrup (if using) in a blender.
2. Blend the ingredients on high speed until smooth and well combined. If the smoothie is too thick, you can add more almond milk or a splash of water to reach your desired consistency.
3. Taste the smoothie and adjust the sweetness by adding more honey or maple syrup if needed.
4. If you prefer a colder smoothie, you can add ice cubes and blend again until well combined.

5. Pour the blueberry almond butter smoothie into glasses.

6. Optionally, garnish with a few whole blueberries or a drizzle of almond butter.

7. Enjoy this delicious and protein-packed blueberry almond butter smoothie as a satisfying and nutritious beverage!

Cucumber Mint Detox Smoothie

Ingredients:

- 1 cucumber, peeled and sliced
- 1/2 cup fresh mint leaves
- 1 green apple, cored and sliced
- 1 cup spinach leaves
- 1/2 lemon, juiced
- 1 cup coconut water or water
- 1 tablespoon chia seeds (optional)
- Ice cubes (optional)

Instructions:

1. Place cucumber slices, fresh mint leaves, sliced green apple, spinach leaves, lemon juice, coconut water or water, and chia seeds (if using) in a blender.
2. Blend the ingredients on high speed until smooth and well combined. If the smoothie is too thick, you can add more coconut water or water to reach your desired consistency.
3. If you prefer a colder smoothie, you can add ice cubes and blend again until well combined.
4. Taste the smoothie and adjust the tartness by adding more lemon juice if needed.
5. Pour the cucumber mint detox smoothie into glasses.
6. Optionally, garnish with a slice of cucumber or a sprig of mint.
7. Enjoy this refreshing and hydrating cucumber mint detox smoothie as a revitalizing and healthful beverage!

Orange Carrot Ginger Smoothie

Ingredients:

- 2 large carrots, peeled and chopped
- 1 orange, peeled and segmented

- 1 banana, peeled
- 1-inch piece of fresh ginger, peeled and grated
- 1 cup orange juice
- 1/2 cup Greek yogurt
- 1 tablespoon chia seeds (optional)
- 1 tablespoon honey or maple syrup (optional, for sweetness)
- Ice cubes (optional)

Instructions:

1. Place chopped carrots, peeled and segmented orange, peeled banana, grated fresh ginger, orange juice, Greek yogurt, chia seeds (if using), and honey or maple syrup (if using) in a blender.
2. Blend the ingredients on high speed until smooth and well combined. If the smoothie is too thick, you can add more orange juice or a splash of water to reach your desired consistency.
3. If you prefer a colder smoothie, you can add ice cubes and blend again until well combined.
4. Taste the smoothie and adjust the sweetness by adding more honey or maple syrup if needed.
5. Pour the orange carrot ginger smoothie into glasses.

6. Optionally, garnish with a slice of orange or a sprinkle of grated ginger.

7. Enjoy this vitamin-packed and zesty orange carrot ginger smoothie as a refreshing and nutritious beverage!

Turmeric Pineapple Coconut Smoothie

Ingredients:

- 1 cup pineapple chunks (fresh or frozen)
- 1 banana, peeled
- 1/2 teaspoon ground turmeric
- 1/2 cup coconut milk
- 1/2 cup Greek yogurt
- 1 tablespoon chia seeds (optional)
- 1 tablespoon honey or maple syrup (optional, for sweetness)
- Ice cubes (optional)

Instructions:

1. Place pineapple chunks, peeled banana, ground turmeric, coconut milk, Greek yogurt, chia seeds (if using), and honey or maple syrup (if using) in a blender.

2. Blend the ingredients on high speed until smooth and well combined. If the smoothie is too thick, you can add more coconut milk or a splash of water to reach your desired consistency.

3. If you prefer a colder smoothie, you can add ice cubes and blend again until well combined.

4. Taste the smoothie and adjust the sweetness by adding more honey or maple syrup if needed.

5. Pour the turmeric pineapple coconut smoothie into glasses.

6. Optionally, garnish with a pineapple wedge or a sprinkle of ground turmeric.

7. Enjoy this tropical and anti-inflammatory turmeric pineapple coconut smoothie as a flavorful and healthful beverage!

Avocado Berry Protein Smoothie

Ingredients:

- 1/2 avocado, peeled and pitted
- 1/2 cup mixed berries (such as strawberries, blueberries, raspberries)
- 1 banana, peeled
- 1 scoop vanilla protein powder
- 1 cup almond milk (or any milk of your choice)
- 1 tablespoon chia seeds (optional)
- 1 tablespoon honey or maple syrup (optional, for sweetness)
- Ice cubes (optional)

Instructions:

1. Place peeled and pitted avocado, mixed berries, peeled banana, vanilla protein powder, almond milk, chia seeds (if using), and honey or maple syrup (if using) in a blender.
2. Blend the ingredients on high speed until smooth and well combined. If the smoothie is too thick, you can add more almond milk or a splash of water to reach your desired consistency.
3. If you prefer a colder smoothie, you can add ice cubes and blend again until well combined.

4. Taste the smoothie and adjust the sweetness by adding more honey or maple syrup if needed.

5. Pour the avocado berry protein smoothie into glasses.

6. Optionally, garnish with a few whole berries or a slice of avocado.

7. Enjoy this protein-packed and creamy avocado berry smoothie as a satisfying and nutritious beverage!

Kale Banana Walnut Smoothie

Ingredients:

- 1 cup kale leaves, stems removed
- 1 banana, peeled
- 1/4 cup walnuts
- 1 tablespoon almond butter
- 1 cup almond milk (or any milk of your choice)
- 1 tablespoon chia seeds (optional)
- 1 tablespoon honey or maple syrup (optional, for sweetness)
- Ice cubes (optional)

1. Place kale leaves, peeled banana, walnuts, almond butter, almond milk, chia seeds (if using), and honey or maple syrup (if using) in a blender.
2. Blend the ingredients on high speed until smooth and well combined. If the smoothie is too thick, you can add more almond milk or a splash of water to reach your desired consistency.
3. If you prefer a colder smoothie, you can add ice cubes and blend again until well combined.
4. Taste the smoothie and adjust the sweetness by adding more honey or maple syrup if needed.
5. Pour the kale banana walnut smoothie into glasses.
6. Optionally, garnish with a sprinkle of chopped walnuts or a kale leaf.
7. Enjoy this nutrient-packed and nutty kale banana walnut smoothie as a refreshing and wholesome beverage!

Acai Berry Green Smoothie

Ingredients:

- 1 packet frozen acai berry puree
- 1 cup spinach leaves
- 1/2 cup frozen mixed berries (such as strawberries, blueberries, raspberries)
- 1 banana, peeled
- 1 cup coconut water or water
- 1 tablespoon chia seeds (optional)
- 1 tablespoon honey or maple syrup (optional, for sweetness)
- Ice cubes (optional)
- Granola, sliced banana, or shredded coconut for topping (optional)

Instructions:

1. Run the frozen acai berry packet under warm water for a few seconds to slightly thaw.

2. In a blender, combine the slightly thawed acai berry puree, spinach leaves, frozen mixed berries, peeled banana, coconut water or water, chia seeds (if using), and honey or maple syrup (if using).

3. Blend the ingredients on high speed until smooth and well combined. If the smoothie is too thick, you can add more coconut water or water to reach your desired consistency.

4. If you prefer a colder smoothie, you can add ice cubes and blend again until well combined.

5. Taste the smoothie and adjust the sweetness by adding more honey or maple syrup if needed.

6. Pour the acai berry green smoothie into glasses.

7. Optionally, top with granola, sliced banana, or shredded coconut for added texture and flavor.

8. Enjoy this antioxidant-rich and energizing acai berry green smoothie as a delicious and healthful beverage!

Beet Orange Berry Smoothie

Ingredients:

- 1 small beet, peeled and diced
- 1 orange, peeled and segmented
- 1/2 cup mixed berries (such as strawberries, blueberries, raspberries)
- 1 banana, peeled
- 1 cup water or coconut water
- 1 tablespoon chia seeds (optional)

- 1 tablespoon honey or maple syrup (optional, for sweetness)
- Ice cubes (optional)

Instructions:

1. Place diced beet, peeled and segmented orange, mixed berries, peeled banana, water or coconut water, chia seeds (if using), and honey or maple syrup (if using) in a blender.
2. Blend the ingredients on high speed until smooth and well combined. If the smoothie is too thick, you can add more water or coconut water to reach your desired consistency.
3. If you prefer a colder smoothie, you can add ice cubes and blend again until well combined.
4. Taste the smoothie and adjust the sweetness by adding more honey or maple syrup if needed.
5. Pour the beet orange berry smoothie into glasses.
6. Optionally, garnish with a slice of orange or a few whole berries.
7. Enjoy this vibrant and antioxidant-rich beet orange berry smoothie as a refreshing and healthful beverage!

CONCLUSION

In conclusion, the "Hodgkin Lymphoma Diet Cookbook: A Complete Guide with Anti-Inflammatory Foods and Immune-Boosting Ingredients" is a great resource for people on the road to recovery. This cookbook encourages persons affected by Hodgkin lymphoma to make informed dietary choices that promote their well-being by promoting a healthy eating strategy.

This cookbook's incorporation of anti-inflammatory foods and immune-boosting nutrients is a crucial strength, as it coincides with studies demonstrating that such items play a significant role in aiding recovery and overall health.

The cookbook encourages patients to take an active role in their recovery by advocating a balanced and healthy diet, combining medical therapies with an emphasis on holistic well-being. The dishes presented are not only tasty, but they are also developed with Hodgkin lymphoma patients' nutritional needs in mind.

The "Hodgkin Lymphoma Diet Cookbook" stands out as a practical and sympathetic companion as people begin their recovery journey. It is more than just a cookbook; it is a guide that promotes a healthy relationship with food and encourages people to live a healthier lifestyle. In summary, it demonstrates that making intelligent, nutrition-focused choices can considerably improve one's general well-being during and after the challenges of Hodgkin cancer.

HAPPY COOKING!

HODGKIN LYMPHOMA DIET
MEAL PLANNER

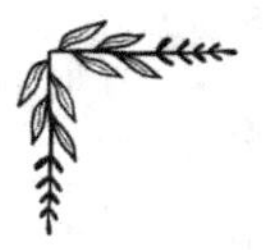

WEEKLY MEAL PLANNER

MONDAY	TUESDAY	WEDNESDAY

THURSDAY	FRIDAY	SHOPPING LIST

SATURDAY	SUNDAY	

Notes:

WEEKLY MEAL PLANNER

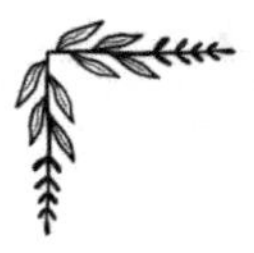

MONDAY

TUESDAY

WEDNESDAY

THURSDAY

FRIDAY

SHOPPING LIST

SATURDAY

SUNDAY

Notes:

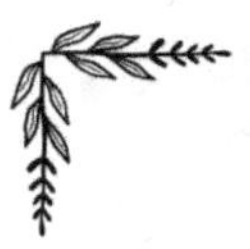

WEEKLY MEAL PLANNER

MONDAY	TUESDAY	WEDNESDAY

THURSDAY	FRIDAY	SHOPPING LIST

SATURDAY	SUNDAY

Notes:

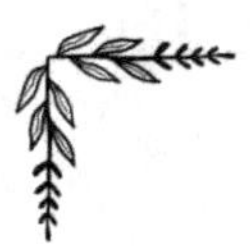

WEEKLY MEAL PLANNER

MONDAY	TUESDAY	WEDNESDAY

THURSDAY	FRIDAY	SHOPPING LIST

SATURDAY	SUNDAY

Notes:

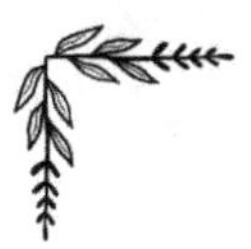

WEEKLY MEAL PLANNER

MONDAY	TUESDAY	WEDNESDAY

THURSDAY	FRIDAY	**SHOPPING LIST**

SATURDAY	SUNDAY

Notes:

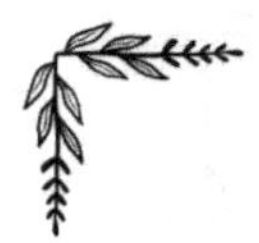

WEEKLY MEAL PLANNER

MONDAY	**TUESDAY**	**WEDNESDAY**

THURSDAY	**FRIDAY**	SHOPPING LIST

SATURDAY	**SUNDAY**

Notes:

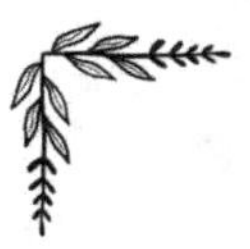

WEEKLY MEAL PLANNER

MONDAY	TUESDAY	WEDNESDAY

THURSDAY	FRIDAY	**SHOPPING LIST**

SATURDAY	SUNDAY

Notes:

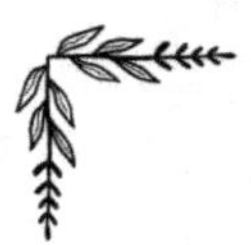

WEEKLY MEAL PLANNER

MONDAY	TUESDAY	WEDNESDAY

THURSDAY	FRIDAY	SHOPPING LIST

SATURDAY	SUNDAY

Notes:

www.ingramcontent.com/pod-product-compliance
Lightning Source LLC
Chambersburg PA
CBHW070919260726
48661CB00003B/759